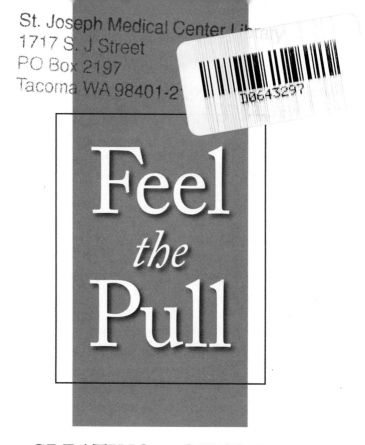

Feel *the* Pull

CREATING *a* CULTURE *of* NURSING EXCELLENCE

Gen Guanci, R.N.

CREATIVE

HEALTH CARE

MANAGEMENT

ISBN 13: 978-1-886624-13-9
ISBN 10: 1-886624-13-5

Printed and bound in the United States

12 11 10 09 08 07   7 6 5 4 3 2

For permission and ordering information, write to:

CREATIVE

HEALTH CARE

MANAGEMENT

Creative Health Care Management, Inc.
1701 American Blvd. East, Suite 1
Minneapolis, MN 55425

chcm@chcm.com
or call: 800.728.7766 or 952.854.9015

www.chcm.com

This book is dedicated to my mother,
whose never-ending support is always welcomed.

To my friends and former colleagues,
Kathleen and Marlene, who made me realize I could write
even when I believed I could not.

To my current colleague Donna, who introduced me
to the fabulous company and people I work with.

Lastly, to Lee,
whose support and sense of humor
kept me moving toward my goal.

Thank you to each of you!

CONTENTS

FOREWORD

In *Feel the Pull: Creating a Culture of Nursing Excellence*, Gen Guanci provides a comprehensive and complete guide to understanding the concept of excellence from both the perspective of award achievement as well as the perspective of deep culture change that supports excellent practice.

Although Gen examines excellence through the lens of nursing, the concepts here are entirely applicable to other disciplines in health care as well as other fields. The language is both precise and concise, making the book highly readable and free of jargon. Gen uses many real world situations to make her points throughout the book. Bullet points summarize processes, and simple formulas explain complex concepts. It is perfect for the busy professional or executive.

Gen creates a pragmatic road map for cultural transformation complete with guides for an organization to follow on the road to excellence. The exploration of organizational assessment is followed with an excellent discussion of how to plan for the change. The discussion on professional practice, empowerment, shared governance and evidence-based practice are of great value. These areas of practice development are often overlooked and yet are the roots of true excellence-in-practice.

This book is in sharp contrast to some other approaches to achieving excellence that provide more of a 'band-aid' than a cure. Following the process Gen has laid out will enable an organization to undergo deep and lasting culture change that will provide empowered employees the energy, courage and will to be innovative and creative care givers. This book is not a 'canned package', full of slogans or catch phrases, designed to merely improve scores or achieve better statistics for some report. The book leads readers on the journey to true excellence in practice.

—*Marie Manthey*

ACKNOWLEDGEMENTS

This book would not be possible without the contributions of the wonderful and passionate team of professionals of Creative Health Care Management. Support, feedback and encouragement from these professionals played a critical role in the evolution of this book.

My sincere gratitude and profound thank you to the following individuals:

Beth Beaty, *Managing Editor*

Chris Bjork, *Director of Resources*

Phillip Schwartzkopf, *Director of Marketing*

Leah Kinnaird, *Consultant and Peer Reviewer*

Marie Manthey, *Consultant, Foreword Author and Peer Reviewer*

Donna Wright, *Consultant and Peer Reviewer*

Mori Studio, Inc., *Design and Layout*

I am so proud to have you as my colleagues!

INTRODUCTION

What is nursing excellence? How is it measured? Why does it matter? What are the essentials of nursing excellence? Where do we start? While many individual articles and books have been published regarding various excellence awards available in health care, there is a scarcity of materials that look at multiple awards side by side and identify the components, or essentials, of a culture of nursing excellence. This book, while not a "cookbook" with recipes to achieve specific awards, looks at the common components seen in organizations that have been successful in receiving national recognition for health care and nursing-specific excellence. Whether you are testing the waters and considering pursuing one of these awards, already on your journey, or striving to implement a culture of nursing excellence without officially seeking award recognition, this book will become your constant reference.

The chapters take you through an overview of several of the awards available in health care today, including the Malcolm Baldrige National Quality Program Award and the American Nurses Credentialing Center's Magnet Recognition Program. As you continue through the chapters, they look at the benefits of creating a culture of nursing excellence, the essentials of this culture, and strategies to facilitate the implementation of the essentials as well as the cultural transformation that inevitably occurs when an organization implements the multifaceted aspects of a culture of nursing excellence.

This book will not walk you through the stages of the application process of any of the awards, nor will you receive step-by-step "how to" instructions. What it *will* do is stimulate your thinking on what it will take in *your* organization to implement a culture of nursing excellence.

As you progress through the chapters and begin to map out your journey, you would be wise to keep the *Power of Five Model for Nursing Excellence* (Figure 1) (Guanci, 2007) in mind:

1. **Educate**

   Educate self and your organization on the measures of nursing excellence (award criteria).

2. **Examine**

   Conduct a thorough gap assessment.

3. **Essentials**

   The essentials are elements of success ... the "must haves." Develop your action plan based upon the essentials and your gap results.

4. **Empowerment**

   Develop programs/processes that support employee involvement and ownership.

5. **Enculturation**
   The essentials must become a part of your organization's culture in order to sustain the award-winning environment. (Guanci, 2007)

The tips, suggestions and tools found in this book are examples of the initiative, innovation and creativity it takes to successfully build a culture of nursing excellence regardless of the type of organization. You will see that it is not enough to simply create a culture that is only "skin deep." Total enculturation needs to occur in order for an organization to sustain the true essence of a culture of nursing excellence.

*"What you get by reaching your destination isn't as important as what you **become** by reaching your destination."*
—AUTHOR UNKNOWN

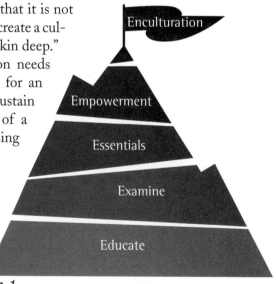

Fig. 1

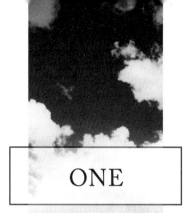

ONE

WHAT IS NURSING EXCELLENCE?

If given the option of eating at a four-star (good) restaurant or a five-star (excellent) restaurant, which one would you choose? It is safe to say that most people will choose the excellent restaurant. The same is true when it comes to health care and employment options. In this day of competition for shrinking workforce resources, in particular the nursing workforce, organizations wishing to stand out are looking at those that have been successful. They are looking at models of excellence.

An online search turns up many, yet similar, definitions of the word *excellence*: "The quality of excelling" (Wikipedia, 2007), "possessing good qualities in high degree" (YourDictionary.com, 2007), "state of possessing good qualities in an eminent degree" and "superior in virtue" (Merriam-Webster Online, 2007). Regardless of which definition you subscribe to, it is clear that in order to be excellent your organization must position itself above the mainstream.

Nursing excellence can be measured by several factors, the most common being results of patient satisfaction surveys, especially as they relate to the care patients received. Others include employee engagement or nurse satisfaction surveys, physician satisfaction surveys and nurse-sensitive quality indicators. While the results of these measures are primarily for internal use, excellent organizations, and those seeking recognition of their excellence, are utilizing national benchmarks as a point of reference.

So how do you validate your organization's excellence? There are many associations and establishments that grant recognition and awards that signify excellence. Awards vary from generic types (such as Best Places to Work) to health care specific (such as the Malcolm Baldrige National Quality Program Award) to the nursing-specific Magnet Recognition Program designation. While the criteria and categories of evaluation for the awards vary, if you were to compare awards side by side, you would see common themes emerging. These are the essentials of a culture of excellence.

Before looking at the essentials, a review of the several awards available in health care today is warranted. Current awards include:

- Best Places to Work (usually business journal sponsored, i.e., Boston Business Journal's Best Places to Work Award)

- American Association of Critical-Care Nurses (AACN) Beacon Award
- Joint Commission's Ernest Amory Codman Award
- Malcolm Baldrige National Quality Program Award
- American Nurses Credentialing Center (ANCC) Magnet Recognition Program designation

Overview of Select Awards

Best Places to Work

Many local business journals have an annual competition for organizations to be designated a "best place to work." Organizations receiving this designation are those that create positive work environments for their employees. In addition these organizations help create a work-life balance for their employees. These positive environments are those that attract and retain employees. This is accomplished through a variety of programs including benefits, organizational culture, working conditions and attention to staff well-being. The process is two-pronged, with the award-seeking organization completing a self-assessment while its employees complete a confidential survey. The employer's questions range from those asking for specifics regarding retirement plans, health insurance, employee education and other organization benefits to questions regarding vacancy and turnover rates. Employees are asked to answer questions such as those related to rewards and recognition, relationships with their supervisors, potential for career growth and their favorite things about the organization.

American Association of Critical-Care Nurses Beacon Award

In 2003 the American Association of Critical-Care Nurses (AACN) established the Beacon Award for Critical Care Excellence. Critical Care Units as well as Progressive Care Units are eligible for the Beacon Award. The purpose of the award is to:

- Recognize excellence in the intensive care environments in which nurses work and critically ill patients live.

- Recognize excellence of the highest quality measures, processes, structures and outcomes based upon evidence.

- Recognize excellence in collaboration, communication and partnerships that support the value of healing and humane environments.

- Develop a program that contributes to actualization of AACN's mission, vision and values. (American Association of Critical-Care Nurses, n.d.)

Applicants for the Beacon Award are evaluated in six categories:

1. **Recruitment and retention** looks at staff satisfaction as well as what the unit is doing related to benefits and employee quality of life.

2. **Education/training and mentoring** evaluates the initial education as well as the ongoing education of staff. It also looks at the mentoring opportunities and the incentives offered for certification.

3. **Evidence-based practice and research** reviews the unit's use of evidence-based protocols in the development of nursing practice as well as staff access to evidence-based practice resources.

4. **Patient outcomes**, the largest category, looks at the overall outcomes of the unit as well as those related to specific disease processes. An evaluation of the adequacy of staffing is also completed.

5. **Healing environment** looks at what the unit is doing to address the stressors related to being a patient in a critical care area as well as a staff nurse working in a high intensity area.

6. **Leadership/organizational ethics** evaluates the leadership style of the unit as well as the support for the professional practice environment. This

> includes the use of shared decision-making processes and individual accountability.

A unit receiving the Beacon Award must reapply on an annual basis to maintain its award status. For further information on the Beacon Award, as well as self-assessment tools, please visit **www.aacn.org**.

The Joint Commission's Ernest Amory Codman Award

The Ernest Amory Codman Award (Codman Award), available to Joint Commission accredited organizations and disease-specific organizations, was established in 1996 to "recognize excellence in the use of performance measures to improve quality and safety in patient care" (The Joint Commission, 2007b). The award (named after Ernest Amory Codman, MD, who is known as the father of patient outcomes measurement) is given to organizations and individuals who implemented a significant performance improvement initiative that was sustained over time. Sustainment over time, or *enculturation*, is a critical factor in this award determination. The three weighted components of the Codman Award decision are:

1. Planning and Resources (20%);

2. Performance Measurement, Data Analysis and Data Dissemination (40%); and

3. Performance Improvement Activities and Results (40%).

For further information please visit **www.jointcommission.org/codman**.

Malcolm Baldrige National Quality Program

Signed into public law by President Ronald Reagan in 1987, the Malcolm Baldrige National Quality Program (MBNQP) is the highest level of recognition an organization can receive for performance excellence. Originally designed for business, there are now five industry-specific awards: manufacturing, service business, small business, education, and health care and non-profit. Health care is the newest addition, having been added in 1999. Each year there can be up to three winners of each industry-specific award. Applicants are evaluated in seven performance categories. Weighted scores are given for each category, with the maximum total score being 1,000 points. A minimum score of 500 on the organization's application is required to receive a site visit. Most past recipients have received final scores in the 700 to 800 range.

Applicants are evaluated in these categories:

1. **Leadership,** receiving up to 120 points, looks at how the organization is led, its responsibilities to the public and how the organization practices good citizenship.

2. **Strategic Planning**, receiving up to 85 points, evaluates how the organization develops and deploys strategic direction.

3. **Customer and Market Focus**, receiving up to 85 points, assesses how the organization proactively

searches for and establishes sustained relationships with customers.

4. **Measurement, Analysis and Knowledge Management**, receiving up to 90 points, assesses how the organization identifies, collects, disseminates and improves data and knowledge resources.

5. **Staff Focus**, receiving up to 85 points, reviews how the organization is maximizing the workforce's potential, as well as aligning it with the organization's mission, vision, philosophy and strategic plan.

6. **Process Management**, receiving up to 85 points, examines how the organization develops, deploys and improves process management. This category is about process as opposed to results, which is addressed next.

7. **Organizational Performance Results,** receiving up to 450 points, or 45% of the total points, speaks loudly and clearly that the MBNQP is about results. Not only are the organization's face-value results reviewed, they are benchmarked against those of competitors and other similar organizations.

In 2002, SSM (Sisters of Saint Mary) Health Care became the first health care organization to receive the MBNQP award, setting the bar high for other health care organizations to strive for.

In addition to the MBNQP Award, 49 states have adopted the criteria and offer a state-level quality award. These awards, most using the same criteria as the national award, are often the first steps for an organization in its quest for the MBNQP Award.

The journey to achieve the MBNQP Award is a long one, with past recipients reporting that it often takes upwards of seven years to achieve. From its inception until June 2007, there have been 67 award winners, with six being in health care. In 2006, 84 organizations from all sectors applied for the MBNQP Award. Of these, 50% (42) were health care organizations (National Institute of Standards and Technology, 2007). For further information and self-assessment tools visit **www.quality.nist.gov**.

American Nurses Credentialing Center Magnet Recognition Program

Many of us remember the nursing shortage of the 1980s. During that shortage several hospitals throughout the United States were attracting and retaining nurses and not feeling the crunch of the shortage. With sponsorship from the American Nurses Association, Margaret McClure and a team of fellow nurse researchers set out to determine what was occurring at those organizations that made them a "magnet" for nurses. Their findings, published in 1983, can be grouped into three categories:

1. **Administration**, including flexible work schedules, adequate staffing matrixes and career growth opportunities.

2. **Professional Practice**, including professional practice models, nurse autonomy and a positive image of nursing throughout the organization.

3. **Professional Development**, including customized orientation plans, support for continuing education and competency-based clinical advancement programs (clinical ladders). (McClure & Hinshaw, 2002)

Several years later, Marlene Kramer and her colleagues began extensive research and comparison of Magnet and non-Magnet hospitals. Her research identified the following "essentials of Magnetism" (Kramer, 2003):

- Working with nurses who are clinically competent;
- Good RN/MD relationships (collaborative/ collegial);
- Nurse autonomy and accountability;
- Control of nursing practice and the practice environment;
- Supportive nurse manager/supervisor;
- Support for education;
- Adequate nurse staffing; and
- Emphasis on concern for patient.

Others also researched these "Magnet" hospitals and found that overall they had lower morbidity and mortality rates, higher patient and nurse satisfaction, less nurse burn-out and higher levels of professional nursing practice.

In 1993 the American Nurses Credentialing Center (ANCC) established the Magnet Nursing Services Recognition Program for Excellence in Nursing to formally recognize organizations that demonstrated excellence in nursing practice. The early designation process reviewed organizations based upon the *American Nurses Association's Scope and Standards for Nurse Administrators*. In 1994, the University of Washington Medical Center in Seattle, WA became the first Magnet designated facility. Since that time more than 250 hospitals have gone on to receive or maintain Magnet status. This number, however, continues to comprise less than 5% of the hospitals in the United States.

In 2002 the ANCC, "realizing it requires an initiative on the part of the whole organization and a change in its culture, chose another name—the Magnet Recognition Program™. This change confirmed what nurses already knew and valued … it takes the whole healthcare team to ensure good patient outcomes" (Guanci, 2005, p. 227). Further program revisions were made in 2005 so that the designation review process now focuses on the 14 Forces of Magnetism.

The Forces are "those elements that contributed to an organizational culture that permitted patients to receive excellent care from nurses practicing in an excellent healthcare environment" (McClure & Hinshaw, 2002, p. 106):

1. **Quality of Leadership:** knowledgeable; risk-takers;

2. **Organizational Structure:** flat with unit-based decision-making processes; nursing represented on all executive committees;

3. **Management Style:** participative; visible; accessible;

4. **Personnel Policies and Programs:** flexible staffing models; staff voice in development of personnel policies and human resource programs; rewards and recognition; peer review/feedback is present;

5. **Professional Models of Care**: nurses are accountable for practice environment; are the coordinators of patient care;

6. **Quality of Care**: high quality care is an organizational priority; confirmed by outside databases;

7. **Quality Improvement**: staff participate in activities; activities are considered educational;

8. **Consultation and Resources**: peer support; knowledgeable experts available and used;

9. **Autonomy**: autonomous practice and independent judgment are expected; ongoing peer feedback;

10. **Community and the Hospital**: strong community presence; long-term involvement;

11. **Nurses as Teachers**: teaching is incorporated into all aspects of practice;

12. **Image of Nurses**: positive; viewed as vital to organizational success;

13. **Interdisciplinary Relationships**: positive; mutual respect among disciplines;

14. **Professional Development**: valued; strong education presence; career advancement.

Those that have been successful in receiving Magnet designation state that it takes several years to create, sustain and enculturate the systems, processes and infrastructures found in Magnet organizations. For further information and self-assessment tools visit **www.nursingworld.org/ancc/magnet/index.html**.

FORCES OF MAGNETISM	
1. Quality of Leadership	8. Consultation and Resources
2. Organizational Structure	9. Autonomy
3. Management Style	10. Community and the Hospital
4. Personnel Policies and Programs	11. Nurses as Teachers
5. Professional Models of Care	12. Image of Nurses
6. Quality of Care	13. Interdisciplinary Relationships
7. Quality Improvement	14. Professional Development

Fig. 2

Reprinted with permission from Margaret L. McClure, EdD, RN, FAAN, and Ada Sue Hinshaw, PhD, RN, FAAN, editors, *Magnet Hospitals Revisited: Attraction and Retention of Professional Nurses*, ©2002 Nursesbooks.org, Silver Spring, MD.

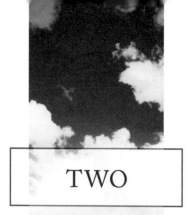

TWO

WHAT DO EXCELLENT NURSING ORGANIZATIONS HAVE IN COMMON?

*Essentials of a Culture of
Nursing Excellence*

As you read the criteria and expectations of the awards in the prior chapter, you no doubt identified several recurrent themes. These themes are what are considered the hallmarks or essentials of a culture of excellence. These include:

- Strategic planning;
- Stakeholder alignment;
- Staff focus;
- Results focus;
- Control over nursing practice;

- Control over the nursing practice environment;
- Rewards and recognition;
- Peer review;
- Use of evidence-based practice; and
- Nursing professional practice.

Whether your organization decides to formally pursue an award (big *J* for a formal journey), or to implement the essentials of a culture of excellence without formal award pursuit (small *j*), the cultural transformation, and the outcomes associated with such a transformation, are priceless.

Benefits for your organization include:

- Aligned resources with strategic plans and approaches (i.e. Six Sigma, Balanced Scorecard, etc.);
- Improved communication, productivity and effectiveness;
- Recognition of the importance of all employees to organizational success;
- Reinforced positive collaborative working relationships;
- Creation of a dynamic and positive environment for all employees;
- Raised bar for improved multidisciplinary patient outcomes;
- Increased marketing advantage;

- Enhanced recruitment and retention of staff and physicians, including
  - Increased retention/decreased turnover rates,
  - Decreased employee vacancy rates, and
  - Decreased "time to fill" rates;
- Decreased morbidity and mortality;
- Increased patient satisfaction; and
- Cost savings related to decreased agency use.

Staff report the following benefits of a culture of excellence:

- Develops organization/unit pride;
- Promotes an environment with increased teamwork;
- Increases autonomy;
- Increases empowerment;
- Develops a culture of accountability;
- Enhances professionalism;
- Increases a safety climate;
- Develops clinical competence of colleagues;
- Decreases burnout;
- Enhances staffing ratios; and
- Ensures a nursing "voice at the table."

The last benefits to look at are those to the individual. While many of these have been identified in either the organization or staff benefits, they deserve repeating here. These include:

- Opportunities to develop leadership skills;
- Opportunities to develop and fine-tune mentoring skills;
- Personal satisfaction and recognition;
- Increased career development opportunities;
- Increased sense of professionalism;
- Return of passion for nursing;
- Decreased burnout;
- Increased autonomy; and
- Increased empowerment.

Some organizations and individuals will look at the pursuit of excellence and say "we are already good." To quote Jim Collins, the author of *Good to Great,* "good is the enemy of great" (2001, p. 1). In *What You Accept is What You Teach* author Michael Cohen says that "the pursuit of mediocrity is almost always successful" (2007, p. 1). The message is clear: If you do not set your expectations high you will never achieve excellence! Remember what Buzz Lightyear said in *Toy Story* … "to infinity and beyond!"

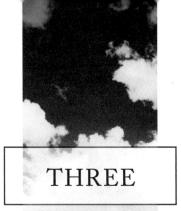

THREE

BRINGING NURSING EXCELLENCE TO LIFE:
Cultural Transformation

There have been many books and articles written about organizational culture … what it is, what it takes to transform a culture and how to sustain that cultural change. Most agree that organizational culture can be likened to the collective personality of an organization. Culture is the key to what can and cannot survive in any organization and even in an individual department or unit. The challenge in assessing and determining organizational culture is that it is unwritten, often unspoken, and can vary from department to department, unit to unit. Culture is developed over time and once established remains relatively stable. Furthermore, culture is strongly influenced by the leader(s).

In his book *Organizational Culture and Leadership,* Edgar Schein characterizes culture as having three distinct levels: behaviors and artifacts; beliefs and values; and assumptions. An apple can be used to depict a conceptual design of these levels (see Figure 3). Behaviors and artifacts, the apple's outer skin, are what are visible and include items such as dress code and workplace design. Oftentimes behaviors are done without the ability to articulate *why* they are done.

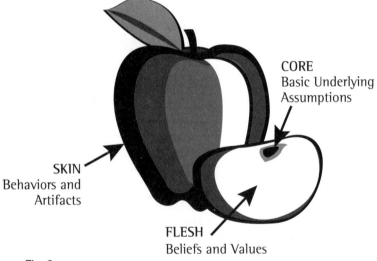

CORE
Basic Underlying Assumptions

SKIN
Behaviors and Artifacts

FLESH
Beliefs and Values

Fig. 3

Peeling back the skin and revealing the apple's inner flesh symbolizes Schein's second level, beliefs and values. These are the foundation of "Why do we do that?" In some organizations there can be a disconnect between stated values and operating values. Asking for employee feedback and opinions and then not acting upon or responding to the feedback is an example of this disconnect.

The third cultural level, or the apple's inner core, is shared assumptions. Shared assumptions are the byproduct of values and beliefs that have been internalized and are now often taken for granted (Schein, 2004). One example of this can been seen in an organization that transitions from an autocratic management style to a shared governance, shared decision-making culture. For years the employees were not allowed to make any decisions. Now these employees are expected to share in not only the decision-making but also the responsibility and accountability associated with the decision. Until the individuals—and the group as a whole—develop trust and new assumptions, they will be slow to embrace the new culture. In fact, they may never be able to embrace the new culture. It is fascinating to interview nurses from organizations who have had shared decision-making in place for many years. They have difficulty imagining *not* having shared decision-making. This is their shared assumption. According to Grace, a bedside RN for 19 years: "I don't think I could work at a hospital that did not give me a say in what I do. Who knows better than the nurses doing the bedside work?"

Factors that influence organizations to change and transform are many. These include external restructuring, a new facility or technology, regulatory demands, visionary leadership, a "burning platform" and lastly, a passion to be better. Extremely poor patient satisfaction results provided the "burning platform" for Baptist Hospital in Pensacola, FL. If they were to remain competitive, this "burning platform" commanded them to undergo a comprehensive organization-wide initiative focused on improving patient satisfaction. Their efforts paid off—Baptist Hospital saw its patient satisfaction scores not only soar but remain among the top in the country. Baptist Hospital is now viewed as a national resource and mentor for other hospitals working to improve their patient satisfaction scores.

Visionary leadership and a passion to be better are among the driving forces behind the growth in award-winning health care organizations throughout the United States. Both the Malcolm Baldrige National Quality Program and the Magnet Recognition Program have culture-related requirements, such as risk-taking leaders and a leadership style including promotion of autonomy and shared decision-making, incorporated in their scoring components.

Jayne Felgen, President of Creative Health Care Management, an international health care consulting company located in Minneapolis, MN, has developed a change model that she calls I_2E_2 (Felgen, 2007). This model consists of four distinct requirements which support leaders in the development of sustained change. These requirements—Inspiration, Infrastructure, Education and Evaluation—are all interdependent on one another. Inspiration (I_1) requires shared vision, a collective purpose and a change at *all* levels. Infrastructure (I_2) is the development and implementation of the structures, systems and processes needed to support the desired change. This infrastructure must include not only the tools but the continuous and comprehensive communication needed to facilitate change movement. Education (E_1) and the development of a learning environment are required to enable employees to develop the skills and competence required for the change. The final E, Evidence (E_2), is the identification of defined and measurable outcomes for the transition (Felgen, 2007). Without measurable outcomes an organization will be unable to validate its success in achieving organizational change. Unfortunately, many organizations fall short in this area. New initiatives are

Fig. 4

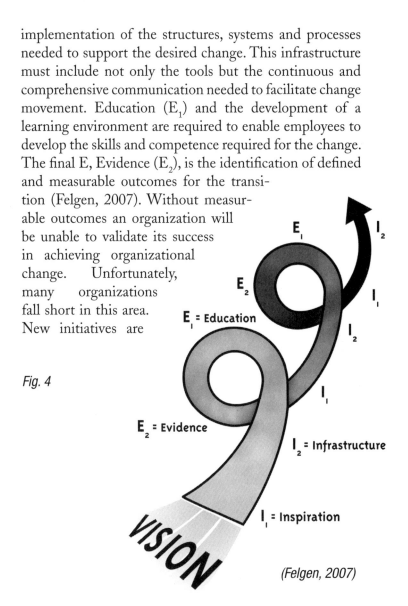

E_1 = Education

E_2 = Evidence

I_2 = Infrastructure

I_1 = Inspiration

VISION

(Felgen, 2007)

developed and rolled out. This rollout is often followed by a brief, informal evaluation of success and then it is on to the next initiative. Minimal, if any, time and effort are given to the sustainment of this change. Felgen's I_2E_2 model (Figure 4) depicts that change is a continuous and ongoing process with frequent reinforcement and/or redevelopment of inspiration, infrastructure and education. All this is based upon the ongoing evidence (outcome measurements) that continuous improvement, or constantly raising the bar, is needed to move from a stand-alone change to sustainment of the change. The I_2E_2 model will move your organization away from a "flavor of the month" approach to a total "walk the talk" or true enculturation of the change initiative.

While planning for change or cultural transformation, your leaders should consider using a Four P approach (Figure 5). The first P entails communicating, to everyone involved in the change initiative, the "Where are we going?" or "Where do we want to be?" Next, communication related to the Purpose must occur: "Why is this needed? Why *this* change?" The third P, Plan, involves the communication on "How will we do this? What is the timeline?" Lastly, every employee must be informed of her role or part in the change as well as how she can help make the change successful. Consistently using this approach has proven to enhance employee engagement.

Picture:	Where are we going? Where do we want to be?
Purpose:	Why is this needed? Why this change?
Plan:	How will we do this? What is the timeline?
Part:	What is the individual's role in the change? How can he/she help make the change successful?

Fig. 5

Proactively identifying and addressing the common mistakes organizations make when implementing change can help minimize and even eliminate change fiascos. These mistakes can include incomplete and/or infrequent communication; not addressing the Four Ps; lack of trust in the process, leader or both; lack of shared vision; and lack of accountability.

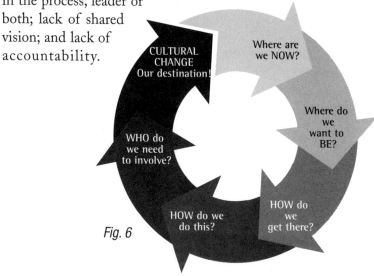

Fig. 6

Regardless of how well planned a culture change is, you must remember that changing a culture is not an overnight process. It is not a "quick fix." Cultural change and transformation can take anywhere from months to years to even decades. After all, it is not just the change you are interested in. It is the sustainment, or enculturation, of the change that is most important. In addition to the enculturation, the change-adept organization is constantly "raising the bar" and challenging itself to be even better.

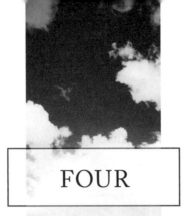

FOUR

GETTING STARTED ON THE
ROAD TO EXCELLENCE:
Conducting an Organizational Assessment or Gap Analysis

As you read the prior chapters outlining the various categories and components of the Malcolm Baldrige National Quality Award (MBNQA), the American Nurses Credentialing Center (ANCC) Magnet Recognition Program, the American Association of Critical-Care Nurses (AACN) Beacon Award and the Ernest Amory Codman Award, you were probably completing a mental checklist. Check, check, check. Got that, need to improve that, need to do that. This is the beginning of your organizational assessment or gap analysis. *Webster's New Universal Unabridged Dictionary* (2006) defines a *gap* as "an incomplete or deficient area; a problem caused by some disparity."

A gap analysis, or self-evaluation, looks at where you want to go and what is required to get there. It is a comparison of your desired state versus your current state. The "we don't have ..." are what some call your pure gaps. The "we have some ...", "we need to improve on ..." or "we have ... in some areas but not all" are also gaps; however, some call these opportunities for improvement (OFIs). Regardless of whether you have pure gaps or OFIs, they all need to be addressed. Because of the importance of a thorough, accurate and unbiased assessment, organizations should consider using an outside resource or consultant to ensure an objective assessment. This outside resource must be someone who has experience conducting organizational assessments. She must also have a complete and thorough knowledge of the specific components and criteria of the award you are pursuing or essentials you wish to implement. Lastly, she must have the ability to generate a comprehensive written report of her findings. Many organizations continue to work with the resource who conducts their organizational assessment throughout their entire award journey. If you think this is the direction your organization will go, be sure to spend time interviewing several prospective resources. You will need to be sure your resource is someone you can work with for the many months, and possibly years, of your journey.

The completed gap analysis will identify not only structures, processes and systems that need to be created and implemented as well as those that need to be strengthened, but also the cultural changes that must occur in order to move your organization toward its goal. Your organization would be wise to keep in mind that it will take much more time to change a culture than to implement structures, processes or systems. Most agree it takes anywhere from one to nine years to change a culture ... never mind sustain this culture change.

One mistake many organizations make when completing a gap analysis is that they do a wonderful job completing it at the organizational level. However, the drill-down to the department, and more specifically, the unit level never occurs. An example of this can be seen in an organization that has a well-established Nursing division practice council that operates under the principles of shared governance. Yet this same organization is lacking unit level councils or has unit level councils on only a few of its nursing units. Whether you call this a gap or an OFI doesn't matter ... it is a deficit that must be addressed.

In order to help an organization determine its "readiness" for pursuing a specific award, most grantors of awards have created readiness assessments. The ANCC Magnet Recognition Program has two such tools available for public use on its Web site. The first tool is the *Organization Self-Assessment for Magnet Readiness.* This tool is aimed specifically at the Nursing Leadership team of an organization. It is set up in the form of statements of what must be present in the organization. Examples include:

- "The CNO serves as an influential member of the organization's highest decision-making body for strategic planning and operations."

- "There is integration of research and evidence-based practice into clinical and operational processes."
- "Decentralized, shared decision-making processes prevail throughout the nursing operations of the organization." (American Nurses Credentialing Center, n.d.)

The second tool found on the ANCC Magnet Web site is geared to the staff nurse. The tool entitled *Staff Nurse Self-Assessment to Determine Readiness to Pursue Magnet Recognition* is a survey that asks staff to respond to questions such as "Does the organizational structure cultivate a positive relationship between clinical and administrative staff?" (American Nurses Credentialing Center, 2007a) Using a Likert scale, staff select one of the following responses: Strongly Disagree, Disagree, Undecided, Agree, or Strongly Agree. This tool is a great way to introduce the various components of the Magnet Program to your organization's nursing workforce.

The Malcolm Baldrige National Quality Program has three tools for public use. The first tool, *Baldrige Self-Assessment and Action Planning* is described as "a snapshot of your organization, the key influences on how you operate, and the key challenges you face" (National Institute of Standards and Technology, 2005). The first section of the tool, "Organizational Description," addresses your organization's health care environment and your key relationships with patients, customers, suppliers and other partners.

The second section, "Organizational Challenges," calls for a description of your organization's competitive environment, your key strategic challenges and your system for performance improvement. If you identify topics for which conflicting, little, or no information is available, it is possible that your assessment need go no further and you can use these topics for action planning. Of the remaining two tools, one is the staff-focused self-assessment *Are We Making Progress?* and one is a leader-focused self-assessment entitled *Are We Making Progress as Leaders?* (National Institute of Standards and Technology, n.d.). Completion of all three tools helps an organization identify its OFIs and will often be the first identification of any disconnect between executive management, other leaders and staff.

The AACN Beacon Award also has self-assessment tools available for public use on its Beacon Award Web site (American Association of Critical-Care Nurses, 2007). Currently there are two tools available, both titled *Are You Ready for Beacon?* One is geared toward adult ICU, and the newest one is geared toward adult progressive care.

Regardless of the award you are pursuing, you should employ an organized approach to your gap analysis and the subsequent action plan. One method is to create a document that lists the specific components, the requirements of the components (the sources of evidence that meet the requirements), and the status of the sources of evidence. Some organizations also find it helpful to then use this same gap analysis document as their action planning tool. By adding a section on who is responsible for each compo-

nent and/or source, as well as the required timeline, everyone can see the big picture (Figure 8). Not only will you
have a measure of where you are and where you need to go,
you will have a measure of how far you have come. It is this
"how far you have come" that will help raise the spirits of
all involved during the inevitable times of self-doubt.

Whatever approach you choose to take with your
organization's gap assessment, you must remember that
this will be the road map for your journey. Just as when
giving driving directions, it is essential that you take time
to ensure the assessment is done thoroughly and accurately.
If you fail to do so, you will end up spending precious time
trying to get back on the "road." Worse yet, you may never
arrive at your destination.

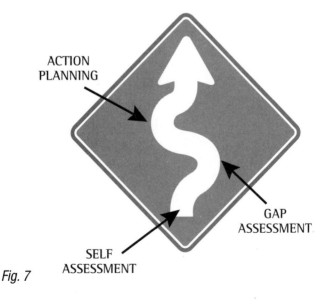

Fig. 7

Creating Your Budget

Like budget planning for a vacation, the journey to nursing excellence needs careful consideration of its budget. These costs must be included in the initial development of the annual budget and not just an "added cost" incorporated into the already developed current budget. Consideration must also be given to the fact that these costs will continue for several years. Many of the costs, if not most, will remain after an organization reaches its nursing excellence destination. Many organizations underestimate the cost of their journey, so be sure to allow adequate time for brainstorming all the potential costs associated with your journey. Cost to consider include:

- **Initial education costs**
  To make an informed decision to move forward on an award quest, your organization's decision-makers must be knowledgeable on what it will take to reach your goal. The costs of registration, travel, hotels, etc. for participation in local, regional and national award-specific education programs must be budgeted for. Additionally, site visits, or field trips, to award-winning organizations is a learning experience that should not be missed—and therefore should also be budgeted for.

- **Organizational assessment/Gap analysis fees**
  Should this gap be completed internally or by an external consultant? Do you have the

FORCE	DESCRIPTION	GAP	SOURCE OF EVIDENCE	PERSON(S) RESPONSIBLE	STATUS
Force 11	*Nurses as Teachers*				
11.1	Describe the process of assessing, planning, organizing, implementing, and evaluating the educational needs of nurses at all levels of the organization.	Yes			
11.2	Describe how the transition of new graduate nurses is facilitated.	No	M/S NN ED NN		
11.3	Describe the orientation and continuing education developed for clinicians, administrators, and other nursing-role specialties at all levels of the organization.	No	Orientation, Charge nurse preceptor programs, leadership development forums and CE programs		
11.4	Describe and provide evidence of mentoring activities at all levels of the organization for both clinical and leadership roles.	No	Student Preceptorships, preceptor program		
11.5	Give examples of organizational incentives (e.g., clinical ladder, promotion criteria, clinical pathways) that promote the nurse teaching role.	No	PNAP, employee excellence fund		
11.6	Delineate staff involvement as faculty/adjunct faculty.	Yes			

Fig. 8

FORCE	DESCRIPTION	GAP	SOURCE OF EVIDENCE	PERSON(S) RESPONSIBLE	STATUS
Force 11	*Nurses as Teachers*				
11.7	Describe all innovative, creative academic practicum experiences that are in place in the organization.	OFI	XX College program		
11.8	Describe the process for assessing, planning, organizing, implementing, and evaluating the educational needs, reflecting concern for cultural differences and language of patient populations at all levels of the organization.	OFI	Annual eval		
11.9	Provide examples of specialty or population-based patient education initiatives conducted, implemented and evaluated by nurses.	No	Bariatric, breastfeeding, Team Steps, heart failure program, asthma program, osteo program		
11.10	Give examples of community collaborative educational endeavors (e.g., guest lectures for affiliating agencies).	No	CPR for schools, clinical\lab instructors for xx college program		
11.11	Provide evidence of broad participation in professional development programs designed to develop, refine and enhance teaching expertise.	OFI	Preceptor programs		

expertise, time and assessment experience to complete the gap analysis internally, or will it be more cost effective in the long run to employ the resources of an external consultant?

- **Award fees**
  Included in this grouping are the fees associated with the initial application, off-site appraiser/reviewer fees and appraiser/review team site visits. Many times the total award fees are dependent upon the size of your organization. The larger your organization, the higher the award fees.

- **External consultant fees (if used)**
  As previously mentioned, a decision needs to be made whether or not your organization wishes to engage an experienced external consultant. This decision should take into consideration the costs associated with time, availability of internal human resources and experience of these human resources to move the process forward in an organized, timely manner versus the fees of an experienced consultant. If your organization does decide to use an external consultant, you can control how much, or how little, involvement the consultant has in your journey.

- **Human resources**
  Consideration must be given to the human resources needed to support the project/

journey. These include an experienced project manager as well as the administrative support individuals needed to support the systems, processes and structures implemented as part of your award quest.

- **Implementation of systems, processes and structures (as identified during your gap analysis)**
Your gap analysis identified what systems, processes and structures you will need to budget for. These could include capital equipment, unit-specific resources, and information technology resources (e.g., more computers so that nurses have ready access to online sources of best-practice guidelines) as well as non-productive time for staff to participate in the systems and processes (i.e., councils). Lastly, do not overlook monies for staff education to support your new systems, processes and infrastructures.

- **Printing costs**
Included in this budget item should be the costs associated with required documentation. Most award grantors require several copies of your support documentation, and many require that this documentation be bound. Additional printing costs include all costs associated with internal materials used for education and informational purposes.

- **Marketing costs**
  Your marketing costs must include the costs associated with before, during *and* after the award journey. How will you market to your staff, stakeholders, patients, community?

- **Celebration costs**
  Included in this line item are the costs associated with winning your desired award and the celebration that follows. Consideration should also be given to additional celebrations in order to help maintain momentum. There are several milestones throughout an award journey that welcome a celebration ... when you send in your documentation, when you complete your site visit or even in the middle of the bleakest winter when your staff is feeling stressed. Celebration costs should include amenities such as food, give-aways, decorations, photos, etc.

- **Award sustainment**
  Many organizations overlook the costs associated with maintaining and sustaining their award. A good rule of thumb to operate under is that all the previously budgeted costs will continue throughout the life of your award. When reapplying for your award, most grantors require that you show verification that you have not only sustained your award status but "raised the bar." This "raising the bar" is often associated with additional costs.

Just as when renovating a home, keep in mind that things often cost more, and take longer to implement, than originally thought, so plan accordingly. Using the home renovation suggestion of adding 15 to 20 percent to what you think you need, both in time and dollars, is a good practice to adopt.

Other Activities

You've completed your organizational assessment and you are creating your budget, so what else can you do to get started on your journey to nursing excellence? Award-winning organizations all agree that site visits are an invaluable undertaking. Locate award winners in your area and arrange visits with as many as possible. Do not limit yourself to the "biggest and best" but also look for organizations that are similar to yours. If you are a small rural hospital, while it will be beneficial to visit a large academic medical center, you may have a hard time convincing your site visit participants that your organization can achieve what the large medical center achieved. Be sure to visit "like-type" organizations. Involving staff in these site visits is extremely worthwhile. The host organization's staff will be able to share their experience with their colleagues and advocate for the pursuit of nursing excellence. In turn, those who went on the site visit will be able to share their experience and observations with their colleagues once they return. The voice of the staff who went on the site visit will foster the "we are all on this journey together" mindset as opposed to the "they (nursing administration) want this."

While on the site visits you may find you form a special connection with a particular organization. The MBNQP Award and the Magnet Program have expectations that successful organizations mentor those pursuing the recognition. Many individuals from award-winning organizations eagerly serve as mentors for aspiring organizations. Seize this opportunity. There will be dozens, if not hundreds, of questions that arise over the course of your journey. Your mentor has been through the process and more than likely asked and answered these same questions. The camaraderie, suggestions, guidelines, tips and how-tos you will gain from this mentorship are priceless!

Other options to increase your knowledge include participation on award-specific electronic mailing lists and support groups as well as attendance at national and regional conferences. Ask colleagues if they know of any award-specific support groups available in your geographical area. While on your site visits, ask the organizations which electronic mailing lists they have found to be particularly beneficial and join these.

Most award grantors host regional as well as national workshops that can increase your knowledge related to a specific award. The MBNQP and the ANCC conduct annual conferences entitled Quest for Excellence and the National Magnet Conference respectively. In addition, they host many regional sessions. A quick visit to the award grantors' Web sites, **www.quality.nist.gov** and **www.nursingworld.org/ancc/magnet/index.html**, will give you access to a host of support materials that you can use to assist you on your journey.

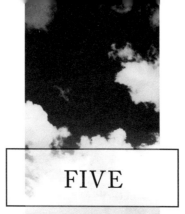

FIVE

How to Get Everyone Moving in the Same Direction:
Strategic Planning and Stakeholder Alignment

Strategic planning, while common practice in business circles, is a relatively new concept for nursing. Organizations have long had annual corporate goals, strategies and plans; however, it is current-day expectation that nursing departments, and even individual nursing units, develop strategic plans that relate to the overall organization plan. Strategic planning is "proactive, vision directed, action oriented, creative, innovative and oriented toward change" (Yoder-Wise, 1999, p. 108). It answers the questions:

- Where are we?

- What do we have to work with?

- Where do we want to be?
- How do we get there?

Strategic planners agree that comprehensive plans follow a prescribed format:

- Completion of an environmental assessment;
- Completion of a SWOT assessment (see Figure 9);
- Development of SMART goals (see Figure 10);
- Development of strategies to meet goals (action plan);
- Implementation of strategies; and
- Evaluation of progress toward goals.

Environmental Assessment

The environmental assessment is a two-fold process that answers the first two questions of strategic planning: "Where are we?" and "What do we have to work with?" In order to answer these questions a review of external as well as internal factors and drivers must be completed. The external assessment includes issues such as geographical impact, demographical impact, competition and political issues, while the internal assessment looks at issues such as the physical plant, human resources, financial stability and resources as well as current programs and processes.

SWOT Assessment

A SWOT assessment is a review of Strengths, Weaknesses, Opportunities and Threats. Like the internal environmental assessment, it too answers the question "What do we have to work with?" The organization's SWOT can be divided into internal aspects (the strengths and weaknesses)

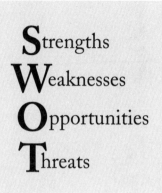

Strengths

Weaknesses

Opportunities

Threats

Fig. 9

as well as external aspects (the opportunities and threats). Some organizations choose to divide their SWOT into positive aspects: strengths and opportunities; and negative aspects: weaknesses and threats. Remember to include in your strategic plan how you will deal with the challenges identified in your SWOT.

Here is one example of a SWOT:

- **S**trength: Committed, hard-working long-term employees.

- **W**eakness: A culture of low accountability or an absence of acceptance of responsibility.

- **O**pportunity: No XYZ award winners in the state.

- **T**hreat: Organization rushes from one project to another without thoroughly evaluating prior projects.

Specific
Measurable
Action oriented
Realistic
Timed

Fig. 10

SMART Goals

Goal setting is the critical component of strategic planning that answers the question "Where do we want to be?" By following the acronym SMART you will ensure that your goals are well developed with an intended/desired target and an identifiable end point:

- **S**pecific
  Something you want.

- **M**easurable
  How much, how many?

- **A**ction oriented
  How will you get what you want?

- **R**ealistic
  Within your control.

- **T**imed
  When will you reach the goal?

An example of a poorly written goal is:
Teach a class on Moderate Conscious Sedation.

The same goal, written as a **SMART** *goal, would read as follows:*
Work with the Emergency Department Clinical Nurse Specialist (ED CNS) to develop and teach a one-hour Moderate Conscious Sedation class in the Spring 08 ED Novice Nurses program.

Action Plan Development

An action plan provides the details and steps to reach a goal. Some call these the tactics or strategies. The organizational assessment or gap analysis sets the direction for the organization's action plan. It is the roadmap of the destination (goal), not how to reach the destination (action plan). Using the SMART goal example used earlier, the associated action plan might look something like this:

- Schedule appointment with the ED CNS to discuss project.

- Independently develop measurable, learner-focused program objectives.

- Independently develop presentation outline.

- Review objectives and outline with ED CNS and revise as indicated.

- Develop session presentation for staff nurse participants.

- Develop session handouts for staff nurse participants.
- Review session presentation and handouts with ED CNS.
- Revise session presentation and handouts as indicated.
- Conduct education session for staff nurse participants.
- Evaluate session using a 5-point Likert scale.
- Revise program as needed.

If you were developing an action plan for your award journey, some action steps would include:

- Hiring or identifying a project director/ coordinator for the specific award;
- Creating a project budget;
- Identifying project steering committee members;
- Developing a timeline;
- Conducting education sessions for key stakeholders;
- Developing action plans for pure gaps;
- Developing action plans for OFIs; and
- Identifying documentation writing teams.

Some may read these action plans and think the plans are simplistic and the detail described obvious. However, for many the detail of the plan is what is needed to keep them on track and moving forward.

Stakeholder Alignment

A stakeholder is any person or entity who has an interest in the activity, goal or outcome. Stakeholders for an award journey include the board of trustees, executive management, leadership team, employees and physicians. Every stakeholder must understand her role in the journey. Roles could include finance approval, the responsibility for the implementation of systems and processes, or the collection of data measuring progress toward the goal. A clear understanding of the goals, individual roles and measurable outcomes must be articulated by every stakeholder. This will ensure everyone is on board. Only when this is accomplished can you begin to move the entire team toward the desired goal.

Everyday Strategic Planning

Every day we engage in strategic planning and key stakeholder alignment in one form or another. Not me, you say? Let's take the scenario of a daughter's wedding. When she became engaged, the strategic planning process was set in motion. First an assessment of the external and internal environments began. The external environment assessment included these typical questions: Who else is getting married and when? When is the venue for the wedding and reception available? Will the venue be available on the desired date? What is the typical weather at that time of the year? Are the desired flowers available at that time of the year? At the same time, an internal environmental assessment is occurring: Will both sets of families be available at the proposed time of year? Will they approve of the venue? What type of wedding can we afford? Who will be in the wedding party? What type of bridesmaid dress will work for Suzy, who will be nine months pregnant by that time?

"A goal without a plan is just a wish."

—ANTOINE DE SAINT-EXUPÉRY, FRENCH WRITER (1900–1944)

You may think the goal for the scenario is pretty obvious, yet it needs to be clearly defined. Is the goal simply that Mary and John will get married? Or should it be the SMART goal—that Mary and John will be married in St. Francis Church, at 2 p.m. on June 9, 2008, by Father O'Toole? Once you clarify the goal then the planning begins (in this case the planning may well have started when Mary was a little girl!).

The action planning for a wedding is so detailed that an entire industry has developed around it. Magazines, wedding planners and bridal shows abound to help those less familiar with the details of a wedding. As the date draws closer, various strategies of the action plan are implemented such as buying the dress, getting the dress altered, choosing the reception location and sending invitations. Simultaneously with the implementation, your daughter is conducting an ongoing evaluation of progress toward the goals and making adjustments to ensure everything will be ready for the wedding.

No matter what type of plan you are developing, there are several key issues to keep in mind:

- Align your plan with the organization's overall plan.
- Identify your key stakeholders.
- Communicate your plan to all stakeholders.
- Articulate your expectations.
- Share the responsibility for attainment of goals.
- Provide written periodic progress reports.

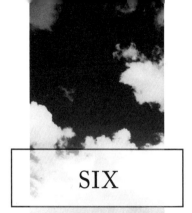

SIX

WHAT IS
PROFESSIONAL NURSING PRACTICE?

We have heard over and over that nursing is a profession. But what is it that makes us a profession? Is it our education? Is it our numbers? Is it the fact that we carry a license? All will agree that no one factor, or tenet, makes a profession. It is a combination of several tenets that include:

- a well-defined body of knowledge;
- depth of education;
- control over nursing practice and the practice environment;
- self-regulation;
- use of evidence-based practice and nursing research;

- peer review;
- the ability to practice autonomously;
- affiliation with professional organizations;
- a system of values; and
- the development of a unique relationship with the patient.

Notice that *caring* and *compassion* are not listed as tenets of nursing professional practice. This is because while caring is the essence of nursing practice, it alone does not make one a professional. The public knows that nursing is a "caring profession," but it is doubtful that they know what it takes to care for a patient. Suzanne Gordon, author of *From Silence to Voice: What Nurses Know and Must Communicate to the Public* (2002), states, "Nurses know that they can and do act on clinical judgment. Now they need to tell the public this" (p. 26). Barbara Blakeney, former ANA president, states, "Nurses do an excellent job of talking about caring and compassion, we present ourselves to the public as people who care—but our failure is that we do not talk enough about the knowledge that backs up the work we do, the reasons why we do those things and how much we have to know to do them safely". We need to proactively address the challenges facing the future of our profession as an intellectual discipline.

Body of Knowledge/Depth of Education

Nursing has struggled for years with the inability, or unwillingness, to define the entry-level education required to be a nurse. Today, we have a cafeteria menu of education choices: diploma, associate degree (ADN), baccalaureate degree (BSN), even a master's degree (MSN) for individuals who are not nurses yet have a bachelor's degree in a field other than nursing. In no other profession are there so many entry-level choices. In 1965 the first American Nurses Association (ANA) position paper called for the BSN as the minimum requirement for entry into nursing (American Nurses Association [ANA], 1965). Yet more than four decades later only one state had changed its nurse practice act to reflect the ANA's position: North Dakota, in 1987, added this requirement to its state nurse practice act. In 2003 legislative changes removed the BSN requirement.

In addition, professional organizations, such as the American Organization of Nurse Executives (AONE) as well as specialty organizations such as the National Association of Neonatal Nurses (NANN) have published statements in support of the ANA position paper.

A review of all health care professions finds entry-level nurses are the least educated. Occupational therapy (OT) and physical therapy (PT) have changed the entry-level requirement to a master's degree. In some health care specialties an aide or assistant, such as the PT aide or OT aide, is educated at the associate degree level.

Linda Aikens, PhD, RN, and her University of Pennsylvania colleagues, whose research study "Educational Levels of Hospital Nurses and Surgical Patient Mortality" was published in the *Journal of the American Medical Association* (2003), compared the three types of basic nursing education programs (RN diploma, associate degree, and baccalaureate) and found a significant relationship between the education of nurses and patient deaths: "Our findings indicate that surgical patients cared for in hospitals in which higher proportions of direct care RNs held bachelor's degrees experienced a substantial survival advantage over those treated in hospitals in which fewer staff nurses had bachelor's or higher degrees" (Atkins & Nygaard, 2003, p. 1618).

The double-edged news is that the issue of entry-level education requirements has not gone away, as many opponents had hoped. The exasperating news is we have missed several "deadlines." In 1978 the ANA created a resolution that "by 1985 the baccalaureate degree would be the required minimum preparation" (American Nurses Association, 1978a, p. 1). In 1982, the ANA again reaffirmed this. Yet with the initial target date of 1985 looming and no significant progress toward adoption of the resolution by the various states, the ANA reneged and issued a new target date of 1995. Unfortunately, that date also came and went. The current deadline is 2010 as the target date for the BSN as the required entry-level education (Barter & McFarland, 2001). If this is to come to fruition, there remains much work to be done!

Many organizations seeking organizational excellence have created on-site BSN programs. Additionally, many organizations have created financial support initiatives, for those wishing to obtain their BSN, that go beyond simple tuition reimbursement. Several award grantors look favorably upon these types of programs.

Certification

National certification also plays a role in the identification of a well-defined and deep body of knowledge. Nurses should be encouraged to obtain certification within their area of specialization. But many ask, "Why certify?" According to the American Nurses Credentialing Center's certification Web page, certification builds confidence in your professional ability. It demonstrates that you meet national standards. It validates your nursing knowledge. It shows dedication to nursing as a profession (American Nurses Credentialing Center, 2007b).

One of the major road blocks or barriers to obtaining specialty certification is fear—fear of failure, fear of not knowing where to start, fear of doing it alone. The following messages were among those written by nurses at the American Association of Critical-Care Nurses' (AACN) 2006 National Teaching Institute (NTI) Certification Celebration to encourage nurses considering certification. Postcards with the handwritten messages are now being included in exam handbooks and other certification preparation materials:

- "Dear Future Certified Nurse, I want to encourage you to study, sit for and pass your certification exam. You will be so glad you did. While I dreaded opening those books again, once I started learning it made my job so exciting. I had so many "ah ha!" moments where I connected what I did on a daily basis to why I did it and why it worked. This exam validates what you already know and already do as second nature. It is hard, and you have to study but it is so worth it. Come join a powerful voice in health care."

- "A certified nurse inspired me to take the exam. I had been 'on the fence' and hesitated taking the exam, even though I had accumulated books and review materials, and had attended seminars for six years. This nurse said to me 'What's the worst that can happen if you don't pass? Nothing. What's the best thing? You validate your incredible knowledge and skills. Get on with it.' And I did. You can too!"

- "I was where you are; you already know you care, you already know you're a great nurse. Prove to yourself and others you can take it a step further and become certified!"

- "You have the courage and knowledge within you. Reach for your dream without fear of failure, but with the vision of satisfaction as you achieve your dream and become a better care provider. JUST DO IT!!" (American Association of Critical-Care Nurses, 2006, p.7)

If your organization wishes to achieve excellence, you should consider programs that encourage and support certification endeavors. Many organizations will reimburse the certification exam cost only after the candidate is successful. For many nurses, it is this initial outlay of the $200 to $400 exam fee that is their deal breaker. They just cannot afford to pay this fee hoping they will pass the exam and then receive reimbursement. The organizations that excel at excellence are the ones that are willing to invest in their employees and pay the exam fee up front. These same organizations do not require repayment in the event the candidate is not successful. This sends a powerful message to the employee: We value you, we are willing to take risks and we will support you in this endeavor regardless of the outcome.

Other approaches to increase interest in certification include financial support for review courses, hosting on-site review courses and even conducting home-grown study groups. While on their Magnet journey, one organization took this study group approach when 11 of their nursing leadership team decided to sit for the ANCC Certified Nursing Administrator (CNA) exam. The group made a considerable time commitment requiring them to meet for one hour every week for 20 weeks. The study group was participant led, with each leader taking responsibility for the review of two or three topics. The organization paid for review books for each participant as well as the upfront cost of the exam. It also supported the group with a hypnosis session to reduce test anxiety. The organization's support paid off: 100 percent of the nursing leaders attained their certification on the first attempt. This was then highlighted in their Magnet application documents as well as commented upon by their Magnet site appraisers. Similarly to programs that support nurses attaining their BSN, many award grantors look favorably upon programs that support professional certification. Indeed, the ANCC Magnet Program's demographic profile requires organizations to submit the number of BSN, as well as certified, nurses they employ.

Continuing Education

Most professions have a continuing education requirement in order to maintain their licensure. Nursing, however, has again failed to come to a unified agreement on required continuing education requirements. Many states have implemented continuing education requirements, but the amount of education varies from state to state. Of those states that require continuing education (Figure 11) the amount varies from as few as 5 hours to a maximum of 36 hours per licensure period. Some states, such as Florida, New York and Oregon, have gone a step further and require education in specific areas such as domestic violence and infection control. Organizations that have a culture of excellence often implement their own continuing education expectations. These expectations are often found as a requirement in their clinical advancement program. Not only do many of these programs require participation in continuing education programs, frequently these programs offer the opportunity for staff to develop and present these continuing education programs. This gives the individual the opportunity to develop her presentation skills and share her expertise. However, it is not the required education that is the hallmark of a professional. It is the constant striving for self-improvement, the desire to learn, the desire to explore new horizons, the desire to share expertise with others that support nursing as a profession.

Florence Nightingale said it succinctly: "Unless we are making progress in our nursing every year, every month, every week, take my word for it we are going back" (1860).

In the remaining chapters we will look more closely at several of the remaining tenets of professional practice. These include the control of nursing practice and the practice environment, peer review, evidence-based practice and finally rewards and recognition.

States with Continuing Education Requirements	
Alabama	Nevada
Alaska	New Hampshire
Arkansas	New Mexico
California	North Dakota
Delaware	Ohio
Florida	Rhode Island
Iowa	South Carolina
Kansas	Tennessee
Kentucky	Texas
Louisiana	Utah
Massachusetts	West Virginia
Michigan	Wyoming
Minnesota	

Fig. 11

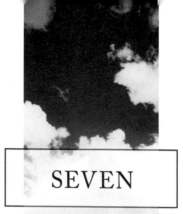

SEVEN

Empowering Professionals:
Control of Nursing Practice and the Practice Environment

For many years, point of care nurses have been told how to do their work, when to do it, and what equipment to use to accomplish their work. More often than not the people doing the telling are far removed from the actual bedside. Materials Management decides which IV pumps to purchase. Nursing Leadership creates the policy and procedure for the IV pump. Staff Development completes the IV pump education—and then the staff rebel.

In the 1970s and 1980s management gurus identified that "companies demonstrating excellence were replacing traditional bureaucratic structures with governance structures that emphasized employee participation and involvement" (quoted in Schein, 1992, p. 33). The age of the employee voice had finally arrived. The word *empowerment* was added to the dictionary and defined as "to give the means, ability, or opportunity to do" (YourDictionary. com, 2007).

The early days of nurse empowerment were rocky, to say the least. Contributing factors included issues such as the social and cultural view of women in the workforce, the dominant role of physicians in hospitals and confusion over what empowerment was. Many misinterpreted it to mean 100 percent control or domination as opposed to having the ability to act (Manojlovich, 2007).

Manojlovich describes three types of power that nurses must have to ensure maximum input into their work environment: control over the content of practice, control over the context of practice and control over competence. Noted nurse researcher Marlene Kramer describes autonomy, the "freedom to act on what one knows," as control over the content of nursing practice. "Staff nurses describe control over nursing practice (C/NP) as a professional nursing function made up of a variety of activities and outcomes. Greater acclaim, status, and prestige for nursing in the organization are viewed as a result, not a precursor, of C/NP" (Kramer, 2003).

In 1985, Prescott and Dennis stated that "nurses should be more meaningfully involved in the running of hospitals" (quoted in Swihart, 2006, p. 5). Prior to the 1980s it was unheard of to have a nurse on the executive management team. Now it is not unusual to have a CEO or COO who is a nurse. A requirement of Magnet designated organizations is that the Chief Nursing Officer (CNO) must sit on the highest level of decision-making bodies. This ensures control over the context of nursing practice. While not a Magnet requirement, a voting voice at these decision-making bodies speaks volumes in regards to nursing's control of the practice environment.

One of nursing's shared governance pioneers, Tim Porter-O'Grady, states that only 10 percent of the unit-level decisions should belong to management (quoted in Swihart, 2006, p. 3). Shared governance, or shared decision-making, is based upon four general principles:

- Partnership,
- Equity,
- Accountability, and
- Ownership.

Porter-O'Grady (2003) defines shared governance as "a structural model through which nurses can express and manage their practice with a higher level of professional autonomy". In the early days of shared governance many leaders misinterpreted it to mean self-governance. Managers abdicated their responsibilities to staff with little support to ensure success. Other managers confused participatory management with shared decision-making.

The differences between self-governance, participatory management and shared governance can be seen in Figure 12.

	Self-Governance	Participatory Management	Shared Governance
Goals	Staff determine goals without input from leaders	Leaders request input from staff Use of input is optional	Staff are give the responsibility, authority and accountability for decisions
Use of input	Can foster a "they...we" mindset	Leader is not required to use staff input	Leadership and staff activities are interdependent
How decisions are made	All decisions made by work team with no external input or guidance	Final decision lies with leadership, who may accept or reject staff input	Leaders clearly articulate the guidelines for the decision (i.e., we have $10,000 to spend on xx)
Presence of leader	Absent leader	Hierarchical leader	Servant leader
Where decisions are made		Centralized decision-making	Decentralized decision-making

Fig. 12

In a decentralized shared decision-making culture decisions are made at the level of action by people in the best position to judge their outcomes.

The outcomes of shared decision-making include:

- Promotion of autonomy;
- Enhanced critical thinking skills; and
- Creation of a learning environment.

In *Shared Governance: A Practical Approach to Reshaping Professional Nursing Practice*, author Diane Swihart defines four elements that are required for the successful implementation of shared governance:

1. A **committed nurse executive** must be invested in process empowerment and must be willing to undertake the efforts necessary to implement shared governance.

2. A **strong management team** in terms of commitment to one another, to nursing, to the organization and to the implementation process must exist.

3. The process can not be implemented if the employees do not have a **basic understanding of shared governance** and if they can not build on that understanding with a working knowledge of what is to be accomplished. There must be a clear destination.

4. The **plan and timeline for implementation** are critical for charting progress points. (Swihart, 2006)

Responsibility, Authority and Accountability (RAA)

In addition to the points mentioned above, a complete understanding of responsibility, authority and accountability (RAA) are required before a decentralized structure can succeed. Many times staff willingly take on the decision-making authority, but they often balk at taking the responsibility, and more so, the accountability of the shared decision-making process. It is leadership's role to ensure staff understand that shared decision-making requires the complete package of RAA.

Responsibility

- clear and specific allocation of duties in order to achieve desired results
- assignment is a two-way street
- visibly given and accepted
- personal ownership and aligned action are evident

Authority

- right to act and make decisions
- restricted to areas where responsibility is given and accepted
- based upon four levels (see Figure 13)

Accountability

- entrenched in role
- reflecting on actions and decisions
- evaluating effectiveness (Koloroutis, 2004)

Levels of Authority	
Level 1	Data/Information/Idea Gathering Authority to collect information/data and provide to another to make the final decision and determine what action will be taken.
Level 2	Data/Information/Idea Gathering + Recommendations Authority to collect information, weigh the options and recommend actions to be taken to another who will make final decision.
Level 3	Data/Information/Idea Gathering + Recommendations (Pause to communicate, clarify or negotiate) + Take Action Authority to apply critical thinking, weigh the options, recommend actions, negotiate the final decision. Includes pausing and collaborating with others before taking action.
Level 4	Act + Inform others after taking action Authority to assess, decide and act. May follow up and inform another of the actions taken as required by the situation.

Fig. 13

In order to move forward in the implementation of decentralized decision-making and shared governance, structures must be put in place. Most organizations choose to create a council structure in which there is representation from areas where nurses practice. In larger organizations this representation could create challenges as the council size could create a barrier to productivity. For this reason larger organizations may choose to have representatives from service delivery areas such as Maternal-Child. This service delivery representation would be the voice for Labor and Delivery, Post-partum, Nursery, Special Care Nursery, Neonatal ICU and Pediatrics. Many organizations go one step further by creating multidisciplinary councils from the beginning or developing plans to incorporate other disciplines in the future.

Council structure should consist of a general oversight council. This is often called the Results Council, Coordinating Council, Steering Council or Leadership Council. Regardless of the name, this is the council that guides the decentralized decision-making process throughout the organization. Membership consists of leaders and staff. After the development of the oversight council, additional councils are developed. The number and focus of these councils are based upon organizational structure and need. Examples of councils include:

- Practice Council;

- Performance Improvement or Quality Council;

- Research/Evidence-based Practice Council;

- Professional Development Council; and

- Recruitment and Retention Council.

(Figure 14, Sample Council Structure.)

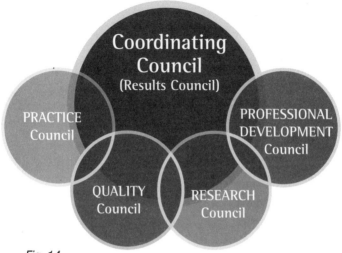

Fig. 14

"A necessary precursor for both autonomy and empowerment is competence." Nurses must own their ongoing development to ensure they are viewed as having expertise as opposed to just experience (Manojlovich, 2007; Kramer, 1993). Years of experience must not be confused with expertise. We have all known a nurse with several years of experience yet lacking the clinical expertise to critically affect patient outcomes. For this reason all council members should receive education related to the council structure and processes so that they may learn new skills.

- Negotiation
- Consensus building

- Meeting management
- Decision-making
- Conflict resolution
- Assertive communication
- Effective discussion
- Facilitation
- Team building
- Change management

The final level of councils resides with the unit. Unit Practice Councils (UPCs) are made up of unit-specific representatives whose role is to identify and address unit-specific processes, structures, issues and concerns. Many units begin their UPCs with the representatives who sit on the larger councils. They then enhance the UPC through the addition of other members. Many times these additional members are identified by asking staff, "Who would you want to make decisions for you?" Some organizations go through an election process. The members of the UPC are charged with the responsibility to communicate and garner feedback from an assigned cadre of fellow staff members. This communication structure ensures input from all members of the unit.

When organizations implement a decentralized or shared decision-making structure, they often overlook the support managers need to facilitate the process. Giving up what, until then, has been control of their units can be very threatening to some managers. Education, support and coaching related to the benefits, outcomes and skills needed for successful implementation of shared decision-making must be given special attention. Keep in mind that shared governance and shared decision-making won't work if the manager won't let it.

There is nothing more difficult to take in hand,
more perilous to conduct, or more uncertain in its success,
than to take the lead in the introduction
of a new order of things.
—Niccolo Machiavelli, *The Prince* (1532)

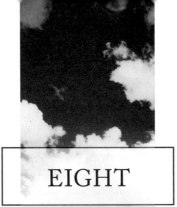

EIGHT

So How Am I Doing?
*Creating Peer Review Systems
That Work*

Many nurses, especially those who work "off shift" and weekends only, are often left frustrated after their annual appraisal. Often they comment, "How can my manager really evaluate me since we never work together?" Nurse managers also struggle with the responsibility of evaluating staff that they have little interaction with. Many managers do make an effort to "work with" each of their staff at least once during the year. This gives them a "snapshot" of the individual nurse's work; however, it is limited. As more and more organizations are fostering the advancement of nursing professional practice, they are turning toward the development of peer review systems that foster professional development and accountability.

According to the ANA, "peer review is an organized effort whereby practicing professionals review the quality and appropriateness of services ordered or performed by their professional peers. Peer review in nursing is the process by which practicing RNs systematically assess, monitor and make judgments about the quality of nursing care provided by peers as measured against professional standards of practice" (American Nurses Association, 1978b, p. 1).

Let's consider an alternative definition of peer review: an active supportive practice to professionally acknowledge and enhance a colleague's performance. The key words in this definition are *active*, *supportive*, *enhance* and *performance*. These are the attributes that must be present in every peer review experience to ensure it is viewed as a developmental opportunity as opposed to a punitive experience.

Most intellectual disciplines, such as medicine and law, include peer review as an integral component of their practice. Nursing, being an intellectual discipline, has identified peer review as a tenet of professional practice. According to research, 95 percent of staff and 100 percent of nurse managers preferred a process of peer review (Lower, 2007). Peer review also:

- facilitates the development of skills for effective feedback,

- enhances the reviewee's professional practice, professional development and education, and

- fosters collegial conversations regarding patient care.

Of the 14 Forces of Magnetism, two specifically address peer review:

Force 4: Personnel Policies and Procedures

Formal, informal, regular and ongoing performance appraisal processes are evident and include self-appraisal and peer review.

Force 9: Autonomy

Peer review processes are in place for all nurses. (American Nurses Credentialing Center, 2005)

The Joint Commission (formerly JCAHO) also advocates for the development of peer review systems to further support nursing professional practice.

The development of a peer review system needs careful consideration and staff involvement. As you contemplate the development of your peer review system, you should evaluate what, if any, peer review your organization is already conducting. You will be quite surprised! Informal *and* formal peer review is already happening in your organization. From an informal perspective, nurses know who they want to, or don't want to, follow for their shift. They know who they would go to for assistance. They know who they would want to care for themselves or a family member. They know the strengths and opportunities for improvement of every nurse they work with.

Formal peer reviews include activities such as precepted orientations, chart audits done by staff nurses, incident report investigations conducted by a nurse risk manager, skill review redemonstrations, mock events, competency assessment programs, national certification, institutional specific certifications such as chemotherapy administration certifications and programs such as BLS, ACLS and PALS taught by nurses.

SAMPLE PEER REVIEW ACTIVITIES

Chart audit

Skills Lab redemonstration

BLS certification

ACLS certification

Precepted orientation

Clinical ladder programs

State licensure

Incident report investigations

National certification

Institutional certification

Competency assessment programs

Fig. 15

The ideal peer review system is one that contains both formal and informal review, is a continuous process and is linked not just to the annual evaluation process. It is the ongoing, informal peer review that will support the development of professional practice.

Like any other process that impacts staff, in order to increase its success staff must be involved in the development of the peer review system. Many organizations utilize one of their nursing councils to spearhead this process. The council is then charged with developing the process, the process guidelines and the tool that will be used. Questions the council will need to answer include:

- How many reviewers will there be?
- Who will select the reviewers?
- How often will formal reviews be conducted?
- How will informal peer review be tracked?
- How unit specific will the process be?
- What dimensions of practice will be reviewed?
- What type of review will the tool utilize (rating scale, open-ended questions, narrative style or a combination)?
- Will the tool mirror the general employee evaluation?
- How will the reviewee receive the information?

There is one concept that must be kept in mind when developing your process ... peer review *must* be safe. Guidelines must be established that ensure safety for each of the following individuals:

- the individual receiving feedback,
- the individual giving feedback, and
- the manager interpreting the feedback.

Elements of successful peer review are outlined in figure 16.

ELEMENTS OF EFFECTIVE PEER REVIEW

The individual is responsible for her professional growth—not you.

Peer review is confidential.

Peer review is a collaborative activity.

Peer review is both formal and informal.

Peer review identifies opportunities for professional growth.

Peer review enhances personal profession growth for all parties involved.

Peer review is supportive.

Peer review is ongoing.

Peer review is safe for all parties involved.

The peer review system must fit your organizational culture.

Fig. 16

Regardless of what peer review process your organization designs and implements, consideration must be given to what education staff will receive in order to ensure a successful process. Most nurses will admit that they feel unprepared to give developmental feedback to colleagues. Yes, they will gladly tell colleagues all the wonderful things they do, but when it comes to advising colleagues of their areas for growth, most nurses clam up. It is the need for these developmental conversations that mandates we educate and coach staff to their fullest potential. Education must include a didactic presentation that reviews components of effective feedback as well as the opportunity to role play and receive coaching.

When implementing your peer review processes, it is recommended that you start out slowly and set up systems that ensure early successes and positive experiences. Peer review, while initially intimidating, fosters a professional practice environment in which colleagues care for the development of each other and coach each other toward their developmental goals. See figures 17 and 18 for examples of peer review forms.

WINCHESTER HOSPITAL
Winchester, Massachusetts
Registered Nurse
Annual Peer Review

Registered Nurse being reviewed:

Unit:

Date:

Describe a situation, or situations, in which the candidate has demonstrated strength. Respond to all three nursing practice domains below. (Domains printed on back for reference)

I. In the caring domain the nurse demonstrates the ability to offer whatever comfort the clinical situation requires or allows. Describe a situation where you observed the nurse exhibiting these skills.

II. In the collaboration/decision-making domain the nurse demonstrates the ability to make skillful clinical decisions based on their prior experiences and skillfully collaborates with patients, families/significant other and colleagues. Describe a situation where you observed the nurse exhibiting these skills.

III. In the clinical knowledge domain the nurse demonstrates expert clinical practice and foresight in the care of the patient. Describe a situation where you observed the nurse exhibiting these skills.

IV. Identify an area, or areas, you believe this nurse could focus on for professional growth over the course of the next year.

Form completed by: (Name & Credentials)   Date:

Fig. 17 Copyright Winchester Hospital, 2007. Used with permission.

FAIRVIEW RIDGES HOSPITAL
Medical/Surgical Services
Peer Review: Registered Nurse

Name of nurse you are reviewing:_____

Your name: _____

The purpose of this form is to objectively assess and evaluate the performance of the above nurse.

Directions: Fill in the circle that best describes performance for each of the items. Include comments that describe observations that support the assessment and provide meaningful feedback.

Clinical Performance	Performance Factors	Comments
1. Demonstrates skills, knowledge and competence in caring for patients.	○ Consistent ○ Inconsistent ○ Not Observed	
2. Demonstrates appropriate action in response to observed changes in patient condition. Initiates action in emergencies. Notifies appropriate person.	○ Consistent ○ Inconsistent ○ Not Observed	
3. Is familiar with and competent using equipment necessary for patient care, including emergency equipment.	○ Consistent ○ Inconsistent ○ Not Observed	
4. Accepts responsibility for completing assigned patient care. Makes appropriate provision for uncompleted care.	○ Consistent ○ Inconsistent ○ Not Observed	

Fig. 18 Copyright Fairview Ridges Hospital, 2007. Used with permission.

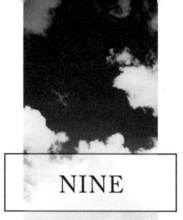

NINE

GETTING STARTED IN EVIDENCE-BASED PRACTICE AND NURSING RESEARCH

Evidence-based practice (EBP) in nursing is the "process by which nurses make clinical decisions using the best available research evidence ..." (University of Minnesota School of Nursing, 2000). However, mention the words *evidence-based practice* or *nursing research* to most nurses and you may see the protective walls or curtains of uncertainty engulf them. Only about 15 percent of health care providers use EBP when making clinical decisions (Cipriano, 2007).

While many think the use of EBP is relatively new to nursing, this is not true. In the 1850s Florence Nightingale examined factors affecting the morbidity and mortality of solders during the Crimean War. Florence Nightingale kept extensive logs of patients' responses to care. As we all know, her findings identified the need for sanitary conditions when caring for the sick and injured. Nightingale disseminated her findings and implemented practice changes that led to the reduction of mortality in soldiers. Her research, entitled *Notes on Nursing*, was published in 1860. The nursing practice of yesterday—"This is the way we do it" and "This is the way we have always done it"—has been replaced by "This is the way it is done … because …."

Many ask, why do nursing research? Why use evidence-based practice? Why not just use medical research? Incorporating nursing research and evidence-based practice into clinical decisions equates to professional accountability to the patient. The use of nursing research and evidence for practice reinforces the identity of nursing as an intellectual discipline and a profession. In addition, it also fortifies the tenet that nurses, not physicians, are responsible for nursing practices. Lastly, to not use EBP is tantamount to negligence.

A review of current literature identifies multiple barriers to the implementation and use of EBP. Lack of time to read research and EBP literature was ranked the number one barrier in a 2005 study (Karkos & Peters, 2007). (See Figure 19.) In addition to the lack of time to read the literature, nurses need dedicated time, free from patient care responsibilities, to develop and implement strategies for the creation of a culture of inquiry and critical thinking. Support from nursing leadership, and the organization in general, is needed in the form of time, finances and resources to sustain a culture of inquiry.

Top 10 Nursing Barriers to the Use of Evidence Based Care

1) Lack of time to read

2) Lack of authority to make changes

3) Lack of time to implement new ideas

4) Unaware of research

5) Lack of physician support for implementation

6) Relevant literature is not together in one place

7) Inability to understand statistical analyses

8) Amount of information is overwhelming

9) Belief that results are not pertinent to current work setting

10) Does not feel capable of evaluating quality of research

Fig. 19 Adapted from B. Karkos and K. Peters (2007). Used with permission.

Nurses' knowledge deficit related to EBP is often grounded in insufficient general knowledge about the research process. This includes knowledge deficits related to the differentiation between qualitative and quantitative research, type of EBP models, and translation of research into clinical practice as well as what resources are available to support the use of best-practice guidelines.

Organizations wishing to build a framework for a culture of clinical inquiry must develop a strategic plan for implementation. Essential to the plan is the development of a learning community via education as well as ongoing coaching and mentoring. While the goal of the plan will be to launch nursing research and EBP, the communication to the staff may very well determine its success or failure. To tell staff they *will* be using EBP is almost certain to be perceived by most as negative. Instead, why not introduce the topic in the form of a study group? This is a safe invitation to those who, while intrigued, may not be willing to announce they have limited knowledge. The study group can cover topics such as understanding the research process, ethical aspects related to research, interpretation of reports, determination of study validity and data collection methods, and a comparison of EBP models.

Many non-academic organizations often say they have no nurse researcher. There are several strategies that can be implemented to facilitate success if this is the case. First, find a nursing research mentor. This could be a professor from a local college of nursing or a professional nurse researcher. If you are a nurse, perhaps the professor who taught *you* about nursing research/EBP would be honored to continue to foster clinical inquiry. To bring the actual conducting of nursing research into your organization, partner with a school of nursing. After all, the school's tenured faculty are required to complete research. Let them know that your organization is willing to support their efforts in regards to access to subjects with the understanding that they will share their results with you. Even better is to ask if a staff member could be a co-investigator on the project. One example is the community hospital that partnered with renowned nurse researcher Marlene Kramer and facilitated research interviews with staff nurses regarding the what, when and where of clinical autonomy (Kramer, 2006).

When your organization is ready to venture out on its own and conduct independent research, consider beginning with replicated studies. This will ease the burden of developing the research problem, question and hypothesis. One recent study that many organizations have chosen to replicate is the effect of hourly rounding of the use of patient call lights (*Meade, Bursell, & Ketelsen, 2006*). Staff nurses see the value of this type of research as it correlates to their daily work.

The implementation of EBP into daily practice requires that staff have easy access to journals, references and best practice guidelines. There are several comprehensive nurse-specific resources on the market today. Many of these products are available through an institutional license that enables nurses to access it via their organization's intranet. Other resources for EVP and best practice guidelines include:

- Registered Nurses' Association of Ontario (RNAO): http://www.rnao.org

- Joanna Briggs Institute: www.joannabriggs. edu.au

- University Health Network of Canada: http:// www.uhn.ca

- National Guideline Clearinghouse: www. guideline.gov/

- Specialty organization Web sites (e.g., AACN Practice Alerts) http://www.aacn.org

- ACE Star Model of Knowledge Transformation (Stevens) http://www.acestar. uthscsa.edu/Learn_model.htm

- Iowa Model of EBP to Promote Quality of Care: http://www.uihealthcare.com/ depts/nursing/rqom/evidencebasedpractice/ iowamodel.html

- Evidence Based Nursing journal: http://ebn.bmj.com

- Centre for Evidence-Based Nursing, University of York: http://www.york.ac.uk/ healthsciences/centres/evidence/cebn.htm

- Nursing and Allied Health Resources Section (NAHRS)-hosted journal club, member websites and other resources: http://nahrs. library.kent.edu/

- National Network of Libraries of Medicine (NN/LM): http://www.nlm.nih.gov/
- NAHRS Task Force on Mapping the Literature of Nursing: http://nahrs.library. kent.edu/activity/mapping/nursing/index.html

Some examples of recent nursing EBP changes reported through professional organizations and journals include:

- Elevating the head of the bed for intubated patients to decrease the incidence of ventilator associated pneumonia (American Association of Critical-Care Nurses, 2004).

- Use of 0.5% chlorhexidine on central line dressing to reduce the incidence of catheter related sepsis (Alexander, 2006).

- Use of two identifiers to reduce the incidence of wrong patient error during medication administration, procedures and laboratory tests (The Joint Commission, 2000a).

In addition to the easy access to EBP resources, a model for EBP should be identified to ensure consistent and thorough evaluation of available research. The creation of a standardized approach will foster familiarity and a level of comfort among staff nurses. Models include:

- Iowa Model of EBP to Promote Quality of Care;
- ACE Star Model of Knowledge Transformation (Stevens);

- The Stetler Model of Research Utilization;
- Ottawa Model of Research Use;
- Evidence-based Multidisciplinary Practice Model;
- Model for Change to Evidence-based Practice; and
- Center for Advanced Nursing Practice Model. (Polit, 2006)

Regardless of the model chosen, there are six major steps to be taken when transferring literature into practice:

- Ask the question.
- Search the literature.
- Critically analyze the evidence.
- Identify the evidence you will apply.
- Apply the evidence.
- Measure and evaluate your evidence application.

The conduction and use of nursing research and the translation into evidence-based practice continues to grow. The Magnet Recognition Program is in part responsible for this since nursing research and the use of EBP is a significant requirement. Regardless of this, many organizations who have moved forward with nursing research and EBP have found out that their staff was "just waiting to be asked." Be sure to celebrate along your journey of bringing EBP to the bedside!

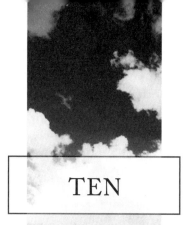

TEN

HOW TO KEEP EXCELLENT NURSES:
Rewards and Recognition

Much has been written about the human need for recognition. According to the Council of Communication Management (2004), recognition for a job well done is the number one motivator of employee performance. While it is the responsibility of leaders to coach employees to their maximum performance, research shows that 73 percent of leaders do not maximize the potential power of rewards and recognition (Council of Communication Management, 2004). This, in part, may be due to the fact that leaders report that they often do not receive rewards and recognition themselves.

Trends Affecting Leaders

There is no doubt about it, the work environment of today differs from that of 20, 10, 5 and even 2 years ago. The trends that affect leaders today are many and complex. These trends can be divided into two categories: those that are business driven and those that are employee driven.

Business-Driven Trends

The nursing shortage, in fact the health care worker shortage, is alive and well. It is anticipated that the nursing shortage will balloon to over one million in the next several years (Watanabe, 2007). All one needs to do is peruse recruitment offers in the Help Wanted section of the newspaper. These ads are full of enticing sign-on benefit options. Options can include four- and five-figure sign-on bonuses, paid relocation expenses, free laptop computers, six-figure annual salaries and school loan forgiveness programs. One recent recruitment ad even offered one year of paid biweekly house cleaning service … proof that organizations are thinking outside the box when it comes to recruitment efforts. All well and good to get employees on board; however, organizations recognized for excellence are going beyond recruitment. They realize retention is actually a higher priority than recruitment.

The Families and Work Institute reports that the turnover and replacement cost of one non-managerial employee is approximately 75 percent of his or her annual salary (2004). Replacement costs for a manager can be 150 percent of his or her annual salary (2004). This means that organizations that experience high turnover rates will end up spending millions of dollars in replacement costs. Therefore it would behoove your organization to focus on your retention efforts to help control these costs.

Another business-driven trend is that technology in health care is moving closer to the bedside and the nursing care delivery team. Computerized nursing documentation, electronic medication administration records and computerized physician order entry systems are leading to decreased "live" communication. The downside of the increased use of technology is that it often leads to a low-touch environment in a system whose consumers demand high touch. Many believe this "tech" approach is to blame for the erosion of workforce communication skills and processes.

The final business-driven trend to affect recruitment and retention efforts is time. Manufacturing has always known that the faster a product is produced the more revenue is made. Time equals money. This is true in health care today. Financial metrics, such as decreased operating room turnaround time, are common goals for inpatient care areas. Also, patient throughput teams have sprung up across the country as organizations struggle to address processes that will facilitate a patient's progress into and out of the health care system.

Employee-Driven Trends

What do the increase in autonomous practice, shared governance and professional models of care have in common? They all share a need for greater employee initiative. Knowing what increases intrinsic motivation is a core competency for leaders today, yet little is done until a problem is identified.

When asked to complete a ten-item ranking of what is important to their employees, leaders ranked "good wages" as #1 and "feeling in on things" as #10 (Nelson, 1994). When employees were asked to complete the same ranking they ranked "full appreciation for work done" as #1 and "feeling in on things" as #2. "Good wages" ranked #5 on the employee list (Figure 20).

	LEADERS	EMPLOYEES
Full appreciation for work done	8	1
Feeling IN on things	10	2
Sympathetic help with personal problems	9	3
Job security	2	4
Good wages	1	5
Interesting work	5	6
Promotion/growth opportunities	3	7
Personal loyalty to workers	6	8
Good working conditions	4	9
Tactful disciplining	7	10

Fig. 20 Adapted from R. Nelson (1994)

Employees have spoken loudly and clearly: They want— no, *demand*—recognition. In his 1994 *Workforce Manage-*

ment journal article, "The Ten Ironies of Motivation," Bob Nelson identifies the challenges that accompany motivation and recognition (Figure 21).

Ten Ironies of Motivation

1) Most managers think money is the top motivator—it is not.

2) "You get what you reward" is common sense, but not common practice.

3) Things that are most motivating to employees tend to be easy to do and cost effective.

4) What motivates others is different from what motivates you.

5) Simple, fun and creative rewards work best.

6) The greatest impact in using formal awards comes from their symbolic value.

7) Recognizing good performance will result in more of the behavior.

8) Managers do not focus on employee motivation until it is lost.

9) It takes less effort to sustain desired behavior than to initially create it.

10) The more you help employees develop marketable skills the more likely they are to stay with your organization.

Fig. 21   Adapted from R. Nelson (1994)

Reward and Recognition Programs

Before any reward and recognition program is established, a leader must know what type of recognition works with *each* employee. Employees no longer want cookie-cutter rewards. They are looking for rewards that are customized and/or meaningful to them. The wise leader will ask questions. Finding out the answers to questions about the workplace is a good place to start. Ask your employees, "What are the things that keep you here?" "What frustrates you so much that you sometimes want to leave?" "What would you do if you were in my shoes?"

Another approach is a "Do More, Do Less, Continue to Do" questionnaire. Once a year ask your employees, "What do you wish I would do more of?" "What do you wish I would do less of?" and "What do you want me to continue to do the same?" Remember, however, that before finding out the answers to these questions, your leaders *must* be committed to act upon the results. Nothing will add to decreased motivation faster than asking questions, getting responses and then ignoring the issues.

Rewards That Work

So how can your leaders reward and recognize employees when they have a limited budget? Keep in mind, employees reported that money was not/is not the top motivator … full appreciation of work done is. With this in mind, your leaders need to be able to engage their staff. They need to be direct, flexible and personal. Keep it balanced. Offer choices. Involve employees in the development of a rewards program by implementing a culture of shared governance. Be timely with your rewards. Create traditions. Individualize your rewards … know what strokes to use for what folks.

A simple yet effective tool for individualizing rewards is the Favorites List (Figure 22). Have all employees fill this out and keep it on file. Now when the time comes to reward an employee you have a reference of her likes. Not only will you end up giving the employee something you know she will like, you will send the message that you took time to customize/personalize her recognition.

Your Favorites List

Just for the fun of it I would like to know the following very important facts about you:

1) Name:
2) Favorite color:
3) Favorite candy or snack:
4) Favorite author:
5) Favorite movie theater:
6) Favorite hobby:
7) Favorite pampering method:
8) Favorite lotions and potions:
9) Favorite restaurant:
10) Favorite place to shop:
11) Favorite non-alcoholic beverage:
12) Favorite charity:

Fig. 22

Other low-cost or no-cost recognition tips include sending handwritten notes. Many leaders already do this, but the retention-savvy leader takes it one step further. She sends the note to the employee's home. In addition to notes, research has shown that retention increased with the use of certain key phrases (Nelson, 1994). While we often say, "You're doing great," increasing your kudos phrases to include any of the following will go a long way: "You are doing quality work on …" "You've made my day because of …" (See Figure 23.) Simply using the individual's name can go a long way in increasing motivation: "Sue, I'm really impressed with.…"

10 Phrases that Increase Retention and Motivation

"You really made a difference by …"

"I'm impressed with …"

"You got my attention when you …"

"You're doing top quality work on …"

"You're right on the mark with…"

"One of the things I enjoy most about you is …"

"You can be proud of yourself for …"

"We couldn't have done it with your …"

"What an effective way to …"

"You've made my day because of …"

Fig 23   Adapted from M. McCormack, Success Secrets

Create theme awards such as the ABCD Award (Above and Beyond the Call of Duty Award). Consider creating a "pass-along" award. Remember Buzz Lightyear from *Toy Story*? He is known for saying "to infinity and beyond!" Purchase a Buzz doll that circulates among the staff. Whoever receives the Buzz award is responsible for identifying the next recipient who has gone "to infinity and beyond." Think of rewards that are visible. Use rewards that let everyone know automatically that the individual wearing the reward has been recognized for something special … buttons, pins or ribbons work well. Create slogan awards (Figure 24).

Possible Slogan Awards

You Done Good

You Make a Difference

Pat on the Back

Top Banana

Thanks for the Memories

The Jugglers

The Big Kahuna

Helping Hand Behind the Scenes

ABCD (Above and Beyond the Call of Duty)

Fig. 24

Consider recognizing individuals outside of your department. This can be easily accomplished by starting each staff meeting with the question "Is there anyone we should recognize?" This recognition can take the form of a handwritten note. Examples could include a thank-you note to the shuttle drivers who drive you to and from the employee parking lot and do so with a smile and a pleasant demeanor. Perhaps an individual in another department just received her national certification. Write her a kudos note. Just imagine how she will feel when she realizes others are aware of the work she does!

For many leaders, *sincere* recognition does not come easily. It is a skill that must be nurtured and practiced. If this is you, make a commitment to find one to three (or more) opportunities per day to recognize individuals. Just be sure it is sincere recognition as employees know right away when it is not! Once you get started it will become second nature, and the sky is the limit. If you need further motivation as to why a leader must recognize her employees, keep in mind the phrase "People do not leave a job … they leave a leader." Don't be that leader! Remember, every leader is in a new job: CRO … Chief Retention Officer!

APPENDIX

AACN Beacon Award Evaluation Categories

1. **Recruitment and retention** looks at staff satisfaction as well as what the unit is doing related to benefits and employee quality of life.

2. **Education/training and mentoring** evaluates the initial education as well as the ongoing education of staff. It also looks at the mentoring opportunities and the incentives offered for certification.

3. **Evidence-based practice and research** reviews the unit's use of evidence-based protocols in the development of nursing practice as well as staff access to evidence-based practice resources.

4. **Patient outcomes**, the largest category, looks at the overall outcomes of the unit as well as those related to specific disease processes. An evaluation of the adequacy of staffing is also completed.

5. **Healing environment** looks at what the unit is doing to address the stressors related to being a patient in a critical care area as well as a staff nurse working in a high intensity area.

6. **Leadership/organizational ethics** evaluates the leadership style of the unit as well as the support for the professional practice environment. This includes the use of shared decision-making processes and individual accountability.

Ernest Amory Codman Award Evaluation Categories

1. Planning and Resources (20%)

2. Performance Measurement, Data Analysis and Data Dissemination (40%)

3. Performance Improvement Activities and Results (40%)

Malcolm Baldrige National Quality Program (MBNQP) Award Components

1. **Leadership,** receiving up to 120 points, looks at how the organization is led, its responsibilities to the public and how the organization practices good citizenship.

2. **Strategic Planning**, receiving up to 85 points, evaluates how the organization develops and deploys strategic direction.

3. **Customer and Market Focus**, receiving up to 85 points, assesses how the organization proactively searches for and establishes sustained relationships with customers.

4. **Measurement, Analysis and Knowledge Management**, receiving up to 90 points, assesses how the organization identifies, collects, disseminates and improves data and knowledge resources.

5. **Staff Focus**, receiving up to 85 points, reviews how the organization is maximizing the workforce's potential, as well as aligning it with the organization's mission, vision, philosophy and strategic plan.

6. **Process Management**, receiving up to 85 points, examines how the organization develops, deploys and improves process management. This category is about process as opposed to results, which is addressed next.

7. **Organizational Performance Results,** receiving up to 450 points, or 45% of the total points, speaks loudly and clearly that the MBNQP is about results. Not only are the organization's face-value results reviewed, they are benchmarked against those of competitors and other similar organizations.

American Nurses Credentialing Center (ANCC) 14 Forces of Magnetism

1. **Quality of Leadership:** knowledgeable; risk-takers

2. **Organizational Structure:** flat with unit-based decision making processes; nursing represented on all executive committees

3. **Management Style:** participative; visible; accessible

4. **Personnel Policies and Programs:** flexible staffing models; staff voice in development of personnel policies and human resource programs; rewards and recognition; peer review/feedback is present

5. **Professional Models of Care**: nurses are accountable for practice environment; are the coordinators of patient care

6. **Quality of Care**: high quality care is an organizational priority; confirmed by outside databases

7. **Quality Improvement**: staff participate in activities; activities are considered educational

8. **Consultation and Resources**: peer support; knowledgeable experts available and used

9. **Autonomy**: autonomous practice and independent judgment are expected; ongoing peer feedback

10. **Community and the Hospital**: strong community presence; long term involvement

11. **Nurses as Teachers:** teaching is incorporated into all aspects of practice

12. **Image of Nurses:** positive; viewed as vital to organizational success

13. **Interdisciplinary Relationships:** positive; mutual respect among disciplines

14. **Professional Development:** valued; strong education presence; career advancement.

Reprinted with permission from Margaret L. McClure, EdD, RN, FAAN, and Ada Sue Hinshaw, PhD, RN, FAAN, editors, *Magnet Hospitals Revisited: Attraction and Retention of Professional Nurses*, ©2002 Nursesbooks.org, Silver Spring, MD.

MBNQP and Magnet Recognition Crosswalk

MBNQP Values/Concepts	Forces of Magnetism
Visionary Leadership	Quality of Nursing Leadership (1)
Systems Perspective	Organizational Structure (2)
Managing for Innovation	Management Style (3)
Valuing Staff, Partners & Customers Staff Focus	Personnel Policies & Programs (4) Interdisciplinary Relationships (13)
Patient Focused Excellence	Professional Models of Care (5) Quality of Care (6)
Management by Fact	Quality Improvement (7)
Focus on Results & Creating Value	Consultation and Resources (8)
Agility	Autonomy (9)
Social Responsibility and Community Health	Community and the Hospital (10)
Organizational and Personal Learning	Nurses as Teachers (11) Professional Development (14)
Focus on the Future	Image of Nurses (12)

ADDITIONAL RESOURCES

Award Web Sites

American Association of Critical-Care Nurses
http://www.aacn.org

Ernest Amory Codman Award
http://www.jointcommission.org/codman

Malcolm Baldrige National Quality Program
http://www.quality.nist.gov

ANCC Magnet Recognition Program
http://www.nursingworld.org/ancc/magnet/index.html

Evidence-Based Practice Resources Web Sites

ACE Star Model of Knowledge Transformation (Stevens) http://www.acestar.uthscsa.edu/Learn_model.htm

Evidence Based Nursing journal http://ebn.bmj.com/

Centre for Evidence-Based Nursing, University of York http://www.york.ac.uk/healthsciences/centres/evidence/cebn.htm

Nursing and Allied Health Resources Section (NAHRS)-hosted journal club, member websites and other resources http://nahrs.library.kent.edu/

National Library of Medicine (NLM) http://www.nlm.nih.gov/

NAHRS Task Force on Mapping the Literature of Nursing http://nahrs.library.kent.edu/activity/mapping/nursing/index.html

National Institute for Nursing Research (NINR) http://www.ninr.nih.gov/

Royal Windsor Society for Nursing Research http://www.kelcom.igs.net/~nhodgins/

Evidence-Based Practice Centers http://www.ahrq.gov/clinic/epc/

The Joanna Briggs Institute for Evidence Based Nursing and Midwifery http://www.joannabriggs.edu.au/

The NICHD Cochrane Neonatal Collaborative Review Group (alphabetical listing of systematic reviews) http://www.nichd.nih.gov/cochrane/

BMJ Clinical Evidence (subscription required) http://www.clinical-evidence.com

National Guideline Clearinghouse http://www.guideline.gov/

Articles

Kramer, M., & Schmalenberg, C. (2004). Essentials of a magnetic work environment, part 1. *Nursing 2004, 34*(6), 50-54.

Kramer, M., & Schmalenberg, C. (2004). Essentials of a magnetic work environment, part 2. *Nursing 2004, 34*(7), 44-47.

Kramer, M., & Schmalenberg, C. (2004). Essentials of a magnetic work environment, part 3. *Nursing 2004, 34*(8), 44-47.

Kramer, M., & Schmalenberg, C. (2004). Essentials of a magnetic work environment, part 4. *Nursing 2004, 34*(9), 44-48.

Kramer, M., Maguire, P., & Schmalenberg, C. (2004). Excellence through evidence. *JONA, 36*(10), 479-491.

Roper, K., & Russell, G. (1997). The effect of peer review on professionalism, autonomy and accountability. *Journal of Nursing Staff Development*, 15(4).

BIBLIOGRAPHY

Alexander, M. (Ed.). (2006). *Infusion nursing standards of practice*. Philadelphia: Lippincott, Williams & Wilkins.

American Nurses Association (ANA). (1965). Education for nursing. *American Journal of Nursing, 65*(12), 106-111.

American Nurses Association (ANA). (1978a). *Entry level education for nursing: Its time has come*. Silver Spring, MD: Author.

American Nurses Association (ANA). (1978b). *Peer review*. Place of publication: Self.

American Nurses Credentialing Center. (2005). *The magnet nursing services recognition program for excellence in nursing service, health care organization, instructions and application process manual*. Washington, DC: American Nurses Credentialing Center.

American Nurses Credentialing Center. (2007a). Nurse opinion questionnaire. Retrieved September 13, 2006 from http://www.nursecredentialing.org/magnet/snsurvey.html

American Nurses Credentialing Center. (2007b). Why ANCC certification? Retrieved July 19, 2007 from http://www.nursecredentialing.org/cert/index.htm

American Nurses Credentialing Center. Organization self-assessment for Magnet readiness. (n.d.). Retrieved September 13, 2006 from http://www.nursecredentialing.org/magnet/forms/orgready.pdf

American Association of Critical-Care Nurses. (2004). Ventilator associated pneumonia. Retrieved July 19, 2007 from http://www.aacn.org/AACN/practiceAlert.nsf/Files/VAP%20PDF/$file/VAP%20Pract.Alert.pdf

American Association of Critical-Care Nurses. (2006, December). *AACN News 23*, 7.

American Association of Critical-Care Nurses. (2007). Are you ready for Beacon? Available from https://www.aacn.org/AACN/ICURecog.nsf/vwdoc/toc?opendocument

American Association of Critical-Care Nurses. Criteria descriptions. (n.d.) Retrieved July 19, 2007 from https://www.aacn.org/AACN/ICURecog.nsf/287342bcf6aa168a88256d7a0079e107/0a5b15123179f47888256da9007276ae?OpenDocument

Atkins, S., & Nygaard, J. (2003). Relationship between patient mortality and nurses' level of education. *JAMA, 290*(12):1617-23.

Barter, M., & McFarland, P. L. (2001). BSN by 2010: A California initiative. *Journal of Nursing Administration, 31*(3), 141-144.

Blakeney, B. Professionalism: An exercise in stretching. American Nurses Association, President's Speech

Cipriano, P. (2007). On the record with Pamela Cipriano, editor-in-chief. *American Nurse Today, 2(4), 26-27.*

Cohen, M. (2007). *What you accept is what you teach.* Minneapolis, MN: Creative Health Care Management.

Collins, J. (2001). *Good to great: Why some companies make the leap … and others don't.* New York: HarperCollins.

Council of Communication Management. (2004).

Felgen, J. (2007). *I$_2$E$_2$: Leading lasting change.* Minneapolis, MN: Creative Health Care Management.

Gordon, S. (2002). *From silence to voice: what nurses know and must communicate to the public.* (2nd ed.). Cornell University Press Ithica, NY. Publisher.

Guanci, G. (2005). Destination Magnet: Charting a course to excellence. *Journal for Nurses in Staff Development, 21*(5), 227-235.

Guanci, G. (2007). Staff development story: Tips for a successful Magnet journey. *Journal for Nurses in Staff Development, 23*(2), 89-94.

The Joint Commission. (2007a). 2007 hospital/critical access hospital national patient safety goals. Retrieved July 19, 2007 from http://www.jointcommission.org/PatientSafety/NationalPatientSafetyGoals/07_hap_cah_npsgs.htm

The Joint Commission. (2007b). Ernest Amory Codman Award. Retrieved July 19, 2007 from http://www.jointcommission.org/Codman/

Karkos, B., & Peters, K. A. (2007). Magnet community hospital: Fewer barriers to nursing research utilization. *JONA, 36*(7-8), 377-382.

Koloroutis, M. (Ed.). (2004). *Relationship-based care: A model for transforming practice.* Minneapolis, MN: Creative Health Care Management.

Kramer, M. (2003). Magnet hospital nurses describe control over nursing practice. *Western Journal of Nursing Research, 25*(4), 434-452.

Lower, J. (2007). Utilizing peer reviews. *Advance for Nurses.* Retrieved May 4, 2007 from http://nursing.advanceweb.com/common/Editorial/printfriendly.aspx?cc=68322

Manojlovich, M. (2007). Power and empowerment in nursing: Looking backward to inform the future. *The Online Journal of Issues in Nursing, 12*(1). Retrieved April 17, 2007 from http://www.nursingworld.org/ojin/topic32/tpc32_1.htm

Manthey, M., & Miller, D. (1994). Empowerment through levels of authority. Journal of Nursing Administration, 24 (7–8), 23.

McClure, M., & Hinshaw, A. S. (Eds.). (2002). *Magnet hospitals revisited: Attraction and retention of professional nurses.* Washington, DC: American Nurses Publishing.

Meade, C., Bursell, A., & Ketelsen, L. (2006). Effects of nursing rounds on patients' call light use, satisfaction, and safety. American Journal of Nursing, 106(9),58-70.

Merriam-Webster Online. Excellence. Retrieved July 19, 2007 from http://www.m-w.com/dictionary/excellence.

National Institute of Standards and Technology. Are we making progress? (n.d.). Retrieved September 13, 2006 from http://www.quality.nist.gov/PDF_files/Progress.pdf

National Institute of Standards and Technology. Are we making progress as leaders? (n.d.). Retrieved September 13, 2006 from http://www.quality.nist.gov/PDF_files/ProgressAL.pdf

National Institute of Standards and Technology. (2005). E-baldrige self-assessment and action planning: Using the baldrige organizational profile for health care. Retrieved September 13, 2006 from http://patapsco.nist.gov/eBaldrige/HealthCare_Profile.cfm

National Institute of Standards and Technology. (2007). Malcolm Baldrige National Quality Award application data—1988–2006. Retrieved July 19, 2007 from http://www.nist.gov/public_affairs/factsheet/nqa_appdata.htm

Nelson, R. (1994). The ten ironies of motivation. *Workforce Management.* Retrieved December 27, 2006, from www.workforce.com.

Nightingale, F. (1860). *Notes on nursing* (1st American ed.). New York: D. Appleton and Company.

Polit, D., & Beck, C. (2006). *Essentials of nursing research* (6th ed.). Philadelphia: Lippincott Williams & Wilkins.

Porter-O'Grady, T. (2003). Researching shared governance–A futility of focus. *Journal of Nursing Administration, 33*(4), 251-252.

Schein, E. (1999). *The corporate culture survival guide.* San Francisco: Jossey-Bass.

Schein, E. (2004). *Organizational culture and leadership* (3rd ed.). San Francisco: Jossey-Bass.

Swihart, D. (2006). *Shared governance: A practical approach to reshaping professional nursing practice*. Marblehead, MA: HCPro.

University of Minnesota School of Nursing. (2000). Evidence based nursing. Retrieved July 19, 2007 from http://evidence.ahc.umn.edu/ebn.htm

Watanabe, T. Nursing shortages fuel debate on foreign workers. (2007, June 17). *Los Angeles Times*, 6.

Webster's New Universal Unabridged Dictionary (2006). Springfield, MA: Webster Publications.

Wikipedia. Excellence. Retrieved July 19, 2007 from http://en.wikipedia.org/wiki/Excellence

Yoder-Wise, P. (1999). *Leading and managing in nursing* (2nd ed.). St Louis: Mosby.

YourDictionary.com. Empowerment. Retrieved July 19, 2007 from http://www.yourdictionary.com/ahd/e/e0118400.html

YourDictionary.com. Excellence. Retrieved July 19, 2007 from http://www.yourdictionary.com/ahd/e/e0262100.html

ABOUT THE AUTHOR

Gen Guanci brings over 30 years of national and international nursing experience and skills to her current role as a consultant for Creative Health Care Management. Her expertise includes the development of strategies and processes to support all aspects of the journey to nursing excellence. She has assisted organizations in their quest for excellence awards, including Magnet™ Recognition and the Malcolm Baldrige National Quality Program Award.

Gen has held a variety of positions ranging from critical care staff nurse to Director of Education and Organization Development. Gen earned her master's degree in adult education from Cambridge College. In addition, Gen holds a Certificate of Advanced Graduate Studies (CAGS) in organization development, also from Cambridge College. She is certified in critical care nursing (CCRN) through the American Association of Critical Care (AACN) as well as in nursing professional development (BC) through the American Nurses Association.

Gen is a member of the National Nurses in Staff Development (NNSDO) and is president of the NNSDO Affiliate–North Eastern Organization of Nurse Educators (NEONE). She is a multi-year invited member of the annual National Magnet Conference Continuing Education Task Force, which is responsible for the selection of conference presentations and posters. Gen has published several articles related to the Magnet journey and is a frequent presenter at national conferences on Magnet as well as a variety of other subjects. Gen is sought after for her ability to take complex topics and make them easily understood.

Gen is passionate about the advancement of nursing as a profession. She addresses this through a wide variety of education programs as well as her through her ability to work with organizations as they develop the image of the professional nurse at their organization.

For additional information on what Gen can do for your organization, please contact her at 800.728.7766 or via email at **gguanci@chcm.com**.

ORDER FORM

1. Call toll-free 800.264.3246 and use your Visa, Mastercard or American Express or a company purchase order.
2. Fax your order to: 952.854.1866.
3. Mail your order with pre-payment or company purchase order to:

   Creative Health Care Management
   1701 American Blvd East, Suite 1
   Minneapolis, MN 55425
   Attn: Resources Department

4. Order Online at: www.chcm.com, click Online Store.

CREATIVE

HEALTH CARE

MANAGEMENT

Product	Price	Quantity	Subtotal	TOTAL
B560—I_2E_2: *Leading Lasting Change*	$24.95			
B510—*Relationship-Based Care: A Model for Transforming Practice*	$34.95			
B600—*Relationship-Based Care Field Guide*	$99.00			
B577—*Feel the Pull*	$24.95			
Shipping Costs: 1 book - $6.00, 2-9 - $6.50, 10 or more - $7.50 *Call for express rates*				
Order TOTAL				

Need more than one copy? We have quantity discounts available.

Quantity Discounts (Books Only)		
10–24 = *10% off*	25–99 = *25% off*	100 or more = *35% off*

Payment Methods: ☐ Credit Card ☐ Check ☐ Purchase Order PO# _____

Credit Card	Number			Expiration	AVS (3 digits)
Visa / Mastercard / American Express	–	–	–	/	
Cardholder address (if different from below):	Signature:				

Customer Information	
Name:	
Title:	
Company:	
Address:	
City, State, Zip:	
Daytime Phone:	
Email:	

Satisfaction guarantee: If you are not satisfied with your purchase, simply return the products within 30 days for a full refund.
For a free catalog of all our products, visit www.chcm.com or call 800.264.3246.